Soft Tissue Roentgenography in Diagnosis of Thyroid Cancer

Detection of Psammoma Bodies by Spot-Tangential Projection

MASAYOSHI AKISADA, M. D.
Chief, Radiology Department
Mitsui Memorial Hospital, Tokyo
Assistant Professor, Department of Radiology
Faculty of Medicine, University of Tokyo

YOSHIHIDE FUJIMOTO, M. D.
Assistant Professor, Second Department of Surgery
Faculty of Medicine, University of Tokyo

SPRINGER SCIENCE+BUSINESS MEDIA, LLC

PUBLISHERS
© First edition, **1973 by** Springer Science+Business Media New York
Originally published by Plenum Press, New York in 1973
Softcover reprint of the hardcover 1st edition 1973

Library of Congress Catalog Card Number 74–2582

ISBN 978-1-4613-5709-4   ISBN 978-1-4615-1759-7 (eBook)
DOI 10.1007/978-1-4615-1759-7

FOREWORD

The practice of medicine changes continually, as science guides the physician to the accomplishment of his objective, the cure of the patient. Study of the history of medicine shows that often a remedy of a disease was discovered before the cause of the disease was known. Often the remedy was unnecessarily complicated, but when the cause of the trouble was discovered, the cure became simple and safe. It is with the better understanding of the true nature of thyroid disease that this book is concerned. Those who read it will be able to make their treatments of patients with diseases of the thyroid more simple and more safe.

Dr. MASAYOSHI AKISADA and Dr. YOSHIHIDE FUJIMOTO have given to thyroidologists a new way of recognizing cancers of the thyroid. Taking advantage of the fact that many cancers of the thyroid contain minute areas of calcification known as psammoma bodies, they have developed a technique of roentgenographic examination of the thyroid that is sensitive enough to show these tiny opacities and to warn the internist and the surgeon that cancer is probably present. There is no question that this sensitive diagnostic test will prove to be of value comparable to that of mammography. And the purpose of all of these refinements in diagnosis is first to warn the physician of the possibility that cancer is present and second, to enable him to avoid subjecting his patient to an operation for a harmless benign nodule which could have been prevented from growing larger by feeding thyroid hormone in doses sufficient to suppress the pituitary output of thyroid stimulating hormone.

The aim of the physicians is to make his treatments more effective and more simple. If he can never employ surgery when it is not necessary and if he can employ it always when it is necessary, he will have attained perfection in diagnosis. I believe this contribution by Dr. AKISADA and Dr. FUJIMOTO is a major step in that direction.

GEORGE CRILE, Jr., M.D., F.A.C.S.
Head, Department of General Surgery,
The Cleveland Clinic Foundation,
Cleveland, Ohio, U. S. A.

PREFACE

This monograph is written not only for the radiologist, but also for the thyroidologist and all those who have an interest in diseases of the thyroid gland. It is generally considered a difficult task to make an accurate preoperative diagnosis of thyroid cancer. This fact is reflected in the conventional policy of removing all the thyroid nodules to obtain histological diagnosis for the final assurance. Accordingly a great number of patients have been exposed to unnecessary anesthesia and surgery, while their nodules could have been left alone with impunity. On the other hand, some physicians consider it best to confine surgical indications for those cases which present a substantial possibility of malignancy through preoperative examinations, namely scintigram, ultrasound scanning, lymphography, arteriography and needle biopsies. However, these examinations do not yield an accurate diagnosis in every case and some are not free from certain hazards and complications.

The technique of neck roentgenography being introduced in this monograph is simple and almost harmless. Psammomatous calcifications observed on roentgenograms of the neck unequivocally reveal the presence of cancer. What is more advantageous is the fact that psammomatous calcifications are more frequently observed in such cases of thyroid cancer in which routine physical examinations and scintigrams give ambiguous results.

Demonstration of coarse calcific deposits is frequently of diagnositc help if combined with local physical findings. When there is an occult cancer less than 1.5 cm in diameter, the demonstration of coarse calcific deposit is often particularly helpful. In 7 out of 11 cases in our series which harbored such small cancerous foci, we could make diagnosis and localization of the primary lesions.

For the technique described here, it is desirable to have a soft tissue radiographic apparatus. However, a conventional x-ray apparatus can also be used for this purpose by decreasing kilovoltage and increasing milliampere-second so that technical factors are adjusted within the range of soft tissue roentgenography.

We are very fortunate to have the opportunity to show the results of our investigation to Dr. GEORGE CRILE, JR. of Cleveland Clinic who visited here as a guest speaker at the annual meeting of "Japan Society for Thyroid Surgeons" in August, 1971. It was a great pleasure that he willingly gave us a foreword for this monograph after reviewing our materials.

This work of neck roentgenography was initiated with the project "Development of Methods for the Early Diagnosis of the Breast and Thyroid Cancers" under the grant of the Ministry of Welfare of Japan. We sincerely extend our gratitude to Professor M. FUJIMORI of University of Gumma who gave us encouragement as the director of the project.

Our study was carried out in the Departments of Radiology and Surgery of University of Tokyo Hospital. We must extend our gratitude to Honorable Professor T. MIYAKAWA, Professor A. TASAKA, Chief of Department of Radiology and Professor S. ISHIDA,

Chief of Second Department of Surgery who constantly showed their interest and encouraged us.

We also want to express our gratitude to Dr. E. TAKENAKA of the Radiology Department, Drs. A. OKA and M. FUKUMITSU of the Second Department of Surgery, Drs. I. KINO, Y. URANO, K. YAMAGUCHI of Pathology Division, Central Laboratory, University of Tokyo Hospital.

Mr. Y. KOGAMO, radiology technician, gave us unsparing cooperation in technical aspect of our work in basic experiments and clinical applications. To Mr. S. HARADA, radiology technician, Miss S. SUYAMA, technician at Pathology Division and other technicians who helped our project we must extend our gratitude.

Mr. T. KIHARA performed a very difficult task of making photographic printings of the delicate psammomatous calcifications revealed on x-ray films.

Professor T. INOU and Dr. M. SEKIGUCHI of Department of Surgery, Institute of Medical Science, University of Tokyo were kind enough to allow us to use their own case which we quoted as the last case report. This was a very interesting case with a long history of giant nodules.

We publish this monograph in English with the hope that it will be referred widely by those who are interested in the subject. We are grateful to Dr. Y. HOSODA of Department of Surgery, Branch Hospital of University of Tokyo and Dr. T. J. IMRAY of Radiological Service, U.S. Army Hospital, Camp Zama, Japan who kindly reviewed our English manuscript.

February, 1973

MASAYOSHI AKISADA
YOSHIHIDE FUJIMOTO

CONTENTS

Chapter I

Introduction

An extensive population survey on the prevalence of thyroid cancer in a non-endemic region of Japan involving 59,106 subjects was conducted by MARUCHI and his collaborators (1971) over a period of six years in Nagano Prefecture. The study revealed an unexpectedly high prevalence rate of thyroid cancer of one per 1,000 subjects in the general population. The incidence among female subjects over 30 years of age was approximately one per 300. Most of the cancer patients incidentally found in their study were unaware of their goiter because of lack of apparent clinical signs and symptoms. This fact explains the extremely low morbidity rate, which is almost one hundredth of the prevalence rate. Actually the thyroid cancer in non-goitrous regions is apt to be neglected by clinicians because of its low morbidity and mortality, when compared to the cancers of other sites of the body generally associated with higher grade of malignancy. However, the follow-up data of patients whose thyroid cancers had not been treated by radical operation showed that the cancer was ultimately a fatal disease in most instances. The results indicate that the principles for the cancer in general, *i.e.*, early diagnosis and proper treatment, should be applied for thyroid cancer as well.

Palpation

In spite of the ready accessibility of the thyroid gland for palpation and study with the use of easily measurable radioisotope, an accurate preoperative diagnosis of thyroid cancer still remains a relatively difficult task.

Time-honored palpation is actually a very important first step in the diagnostic evaluation. With accumulation of experience, the amount of information obtainable by palpation would certainly increase. However, it must be recognized that palpation has its own limitations in several aspects. The physical signs suggesting the presence of malignant tumors, such as hard nodule, fixation to the surrounding structures, and irregular surface of the nodule, are not necessarily pathognomonic of thyroid cancer. Such findings are often seen in cases of calcified benign nodules, benign cystic nodules having had a recent attack of intranodular bleeding and in some instances of subacute or chronic thyroiditis.

A highly experienced physician can occasionally detect a thyroid cancer as small as 1 cm in diameter or even smaller simply by using his well-trained fingers, but when the cancer is located deeply within the lobe, its detection is extremely difficult. The primary cancer is often unpalpable even by a very careful examination with the prior knowledge of a pathological report indicating positive metastasis in the biopsied cervical lymph nodes. Most physicians probably have encountered patients with the clinically apparent blood-born metastases in remote areas without a palpable primary tumor in the neck.

On the other hand, when a thyroid cancer takes the form of a large, firm nodule, differentiation from a benign lesion is very difficult so long as the lesion is confined within the capsule of the thyroid and is readily movable with its smooth, round surface. When a small carcinoma of the thyroid is present along with single or multiple benign nodules or within a firm goiter affected by subacute or chronic thyroiditis, its detection by palpation is extremely difficult or almost impossible.

Routine Roentgenography

Routine roentgenography of the neck has been used as one of the diagnostic tools, but contributed relatively little to the evaluation of thyroid nodule for malignancy. Displacement or compression of the trachea and esophagus can be observed on the standard lateral and antero-posterior views. RITVO (1951) and ERAZO and WAHNER (1966) have attempted to correlate these roentgenographic findings with thyroid carcinoma. But, as SCHEIN and his collaborators (1956) pointed out, this method is unreliable and not infrequently misleading. Simple displacement or even indentation is not viewed as a definitive sign of malignancy. Only clear evidence of invasion indicates the presence of thyroid cancer, which is better demonstrated by tomography than plain roentgenography. For the examination of esophagus, barium swallow is needed.

Recently several attempts have been made to obtain more reliable and reproducible findings. These include scintiscanning with radioiodine, angiography, ultrasound scanning and thyroid lymphography. Detailed review of these diagnostic procedures seems to be beyond the scope of this book, and only comments based on our experience with them will be briefly described.

Scintiscanning

Thyroid scintiscanning by use of a radioisotope can provide a great deal of information regarding the location, size, shape and function of the gland. In general, thyroid cancers are shown on the scintigram as areas of decreased activity in comparison to the normal thyroid tissue. When a nodule is demonstrated as "hot", the possibility of cancer is quite remote. From these findings, the policy ensues that all the "cold" nodules should be removed, because the possibility of cancer cannot be ruled out. If this policy is strictly adopted, a fairly large number of patients with benign nodules would undergo unnecessary operation.

It should be kept in mind, however, that carcinoma of the thyroid less than 1.5 cm in diameter cannot be demonstrated as a cold nodule on the scintigram. Recently several investigations have been performed in order to obtain positive scans at the sites of thyroid cancers by use of ^{131}Cs or ^{67}Ga citrate, but the results thus far have not been satisfactory for routine laboratory work.

Angiography

Angiographic diagnosis of benign and malignant tumors of the thyroid was first reported by BOBBIO and his collaborators in 1959. DJINDJIAN and DORLAND (1963) performed angiographic studies of the thyroid by opacification of the inferior thyroid artery. In Japan, ENDO et al. (1968) and TAKAHASHI et al. (1969) have established the successful angiographic technique in this field. The former used a percutaneous direct puncture of the common carotid artery and the latter tried to visualize both superior and inferior thyroid arteries by a percutaneous catheter technique via the femoral or axillary artery. With these techniques, both groups have succeeded to make correct diagnoses in 90% of the patients. Thyroid cancer showed tumor vessels and irregular, ragged tumor stains. Adenomas presented as homogenous, smooth stains without tumor vessels or as poorly vascularized masses. Thyroid carcinoma as small as 1 cm in diameter was demonstrated on the angiogram by the presence of irregular tumor vessels and tumor stain.

Thus the results are excellent, but the routine use of the technique for all the patients with thyroid nodules is debatable because of its complexity and the skills required.

Ultrasound Scanning

Ultrasound scanning of the thyroid gland was developed in 1967 by one of the authors (Y. F.) and his collaborators as a new diagnostic approach to evaluate the nature and structure of thyroid nodules. Recently THIJS (1971) also reported the diagnostic usefulness of the technique. The examination is done by B mode. It is simple and harmless, and takes only 5 to 10 minutes per patient. This method is extremely useful in differentiating a cystic nodule from a solid one. If a nodule is shown cystic on the ultrasound scanning and physical examination confirms it to be a round, readily movable nodule, then aspiration of fluid accompanied by conservative follow-up is the treatment of choice. Thus, we can avoid unnecessary surgery in those harmless benign nodules which have already undergone cystic degeneration. Only those nodules which are shown to be solid on the scan are considered for surgery. In this latter group, clear distinction between benign and malignant lesions is impossible by this technique, although a heavily spotted pattern is more frequently observed in malignant tumors, namely in 65% of 49 cases, and less frequently in benign nodules, in 22% of 72 cases in the authors' series.

Thyroid Lymphography

Thyroid lymphography was developed by MATOBA and KIKUCHI in 1969, as a new technique for visualization of the thyroid and cervical lymph nodes. This is done simply by injecting percutaneously 2 ml of Lipiodol Ultra-Fluid* into the thyroid gland. Ten minutes later the lobe on the side of injection is completely outlined and 24 hours later its regional lymph nodes are visualized. In the normal thyroid, the lobules are visualized as a fine net-work. The area occupied by a benign nodule is demonstrated as a clear-cut defect and in the case of cancer the area is shown as an irregularly outlined defect. This simple technique has been widely adopted in many clinics in our country and has been highly reliable.

ROENTGENOGRAPHIC DEMONSTRATION OF PSAMMOMA BODIES

It appears that thus far routine roentgenography of the neck has contributed little in the evaluation of thyroid cancers, because the diagnosis of malignancy can only be made with certainty when there is frank evidence of either invasion at the site of the primary cancer or metastasis in the lung or bones, and thus the disease is often too advanced for curative resection. Recently several radiologists have focused their attention on one more sign of thyroid cancer, *i.e.*, radiological demonstration of psammoma bodies.

Psammoma Bodies and Thyroid Cancer

It is a well known fact that psammoma bodies are frequently associated with carcinoma of the thyroid. The bodies are round, basophilic, concentrically laminated structures with diameters varying from 10 to 100 microns. They are also called microliths or calcospherites. These characteristic spherical calcifications in the papillary tumor of the thyroid were first described by PAYR and MARTINA in 1906. KLINCK (1949) was the first to emphasize their occurrence in the thyroid carcinoma and stated that

---

* Lipiodol Ultra-Fluid: Laboratoires Andre Guerbet, Paris, France

when they were found a meticulous search should be made for a primary carcinoma of the thyroid gland. In histologic studies, the occurrence of psammoma bodies in the thyroid cancers is variable according to the investigators, but roughly estimated about 50%. The more important fact is that psammoma bodies are only very rarely present in non-cancerous thyroid glands.

In the series of KLINCK and WINSHIP reported in 1959, 48% of a total of 473 thyroid cancers contained psammoma bodies, whereas only one non-toxic nodular goiter contained psammoma bodies out of 2,153 noncancerous thyroids. BATSAKIS, NISHIYAMA and RICH (1960) reported that in a study of 819 surgical specimens of the thyroid, psammoma bodies were found in 94, or 11.4%. Among the 207 carcinomas in this group, psammoma bodies were found in 40.5%. On the contrary, in benign conditions of the thyroid, the occurrence of psammoma bodies was only 1.6%. In the series of MARGOLIN, WINFIELD and STEINBACH (1967), psammoma bodies were found in 10 of 20 cancers and in 2 of 82 benign lesions. HIGUCHI and his collaborators (1969) reported that the bodies were found in 38 of 55 papillary carcinomas, in 3 of 18 follicular carcinomas and in only one of 33 benign nodules. As will be stated later, the authors' series revealed that psammoma bodies were present in 59% of 100 cancers and in only 2% of 98 benign nodules. All these data indicate that psammoma bodies in thyroid cancer can serve as a diagnostic aid.

In fact several pathologists believe that psammoma bodies are almost pathognomonic of thyroid carcinoma. The presence of psammoma bodies in a needle biopsy specimen from a gland clinically thought to be the seat of thyroiditis led CRILE and FISHER (1953) to suspect the presence of cancer. UNDERWOOD, ACKERMAN and ECKERT (1958) wrote that the presence of psammoma bodies in frozen sections was helpful to the pathologist in reaching a correct diagnosis.

If psammoma bodies could be demonstrated in roentgenograms of the neck, it would be of interest to the radiologist as well as the pathologist.

Psammoma Bodies on Neck Roentgenogram

Although abnormal calcific deposits within the thyroid gland have long been observed in standard roentgenograms of the neck, they have generally been interpreted as representing degenerative benign nodules.

In 1958, HOLTZ and POWERS first reported the clinical importance of the roentgenographic demonstration of psammoma bodies. They studied 53 patients with histologically proven papillary carcinoma seen in a 10 year period. Twelve of these 53 patients had psammoma bodies on histologic sections. Of these 12 patients, 3 showed calcific shadows on the roentgenograms thought to be typical of psammoma bodies. Although their report was a short one presenting only one case in whom a preoperative diagnosis of papillary carcinoma could be made by the roentgenographic demonstration of psammomatous calcification, they were truely pioneers in this field. They proposed criteria by which the calcific deposits in benign nodules could be distinguished roentgenologically from malignant calcifications. They also suggested the usefulness of detailed roentgen study which optimally consisted of antero-posterior, lateral and oblique views using soft tissue technique.

SEGAL, ZUCKERMAN and FRIEDMAN (1960), who had been using the technique of soft-tissue roentgenography in diagnostic mammography, began to apply the method to lesions of the thyroid in November, 1958. Three views were taken and an extension cone was used. Technical factors used were: 54 kV, 40 mAs, non-Bucky and 180 cm distance for the lateral view; 54 kV, 50 mAs, Bucky and 100 cm distance for the tangential view; and

55 kV, 50 mAs, Bucky and 100 cm distance for the anteroposterior view. The criteria they derived incidentally agreed with those of HOLTZ and POWERS in all essentials. Namely, as criteria for malignant lesions, the roentgenograms must show the bodies to be poorly marginated, hazy, not densely calcific, about equal in size, and usually grouped in streaks or in a nebular formation within a well-limited area that does not have a calcific rim. In contrast, the calcifications appearing in benign lesions are usually densely calcified, sharply defined, well marginated, and varying in size. Usually they are haphazardly or individually spaced, but if they are grouped the area most often has a surrounding calcific rim. SEGAL et al. obtained preoperative roentgenograms cf the neck of 29 patients with thyroid masses and reported the results in 1960. Six patients proved to have carcinoma of the thyroid, three of whom showed psammomatous calcification on roentgenograms and presented psammoma bodies on microscopic sections. The carcinomas in these three patients were all of papillary variety. There were no false positive results in the remaining 23 patients with benign lesions.

FOURNIER and JOUVE-FOURNIER (1962) performed roentgenograms of the neck applying the mammography technique and considered the psammomatous calcification as diagnostic of thyroid cancer.

Gasquet, GÉRALD-MARCHANT, MARKOVITS and TUBIANA (1963) performed 450 radiographs of the thyroid gland during a period of two years and two months at Institute Gustave-Roussy. They employed oblique and lateral projections of the neck on industrial film without screens. Eighty-eight patients were operated upon. Of the 28 proven carcinomas, 10 showed psammomatous calcification on the neck roentgenograms. No false positive results were obtained in the 60 patients with benign conditions. Criteria for roentgenographic differentiation of calcific deposits were the same as proposed by the previously cited three groups of authors. The results were correlated with the roentgen appearance of the excised specimens. The latter showed one more positive instance in the group of papillary caricinoma and one less positive instance in the group of follicular carcinoma, thus resulting in the same positive incidence as for the presence of psammoma bodies.

HIGUCHI and his collaborators (1969) and ITO and HIGASHI (1965, 1969) in Japan have employed roentgenographic demonstration of intrathyroidal calcification as one of the routine diagnostic procedures. HIGUCHI used an industrial type of film in his later study.

ITO and HIGASHI have taken two views routinely with the following technical factors: 65 kVp, 100 mA, 0.25 sec., 2 m, Bucky (5: 1) and HS-type of screen for the antero-posterior view; and 65 kVp, 100 mA, 0.12 sec., 2 m, non-Bucky and HS-type of screen for the lateral view. They obtained neck roentgenograms in non-consecutive patients with thyroid nodules and the roentgenographic findings of calcification were classified into three patterns: a) coarse amorphous or circular pattern, b) nebular pattern, and c) irregular aggregation of numerous fine grain deposits and larger punctate deposits. These roentgenologic patterns were correlated with the histological diagnoses. The first pattern was seen in 2 cancers and 33 benign diseases, the second pattern was seen in 43 cancers and 2 benign diseases and the last pattern was observed in 28 cancers and 5 benign nodules. Thus the authors stressed the diagnostic importance of the latter two patterns as roentgenologic signs indicating the presence of thyroid cancer, recognizing that occasional false positives would occur because of the use of standard roentgenography.

WATANABE, MAKIUCHI, SATO and FURIHATA (1970) reported their experience over a three-year period on roentgenography of the neck. Two views, antero-posterior and lateral, were obtained with the following technical factors: 120 kV, 50 mA for the former and

50 kV, 100 mA for the latter.   Unfortunately no soft-tissue roentgenography was utilized.   Of 33 cancer patients, 23 presented psammomatous calcification and one showed
merely coarse calcification on the roentgenograms.   On the other hand, of 27 adenomas,
5 showed psammomatous calcification and 10 showed coarse calcification.

MARGOLIN and STEINBACH (1968) were critical to all the previous investigations, because
no soft tissue roentgenography was performed with strict adherence to the principles de-
signed to provide optimal contrast and detail.   MARGOLIN and STEINBACH employed
equipment routinely used for mammography, and took a lateral view with the following
technical factors: 48 kV, 300 mA, 3 sec., 28 inches target-to-film distance, no filtration.
The oblique view utilized the following factors: 56 kV, 300 mA, 3 sec., 26 inches target-
to-film distance.   A cylinder cone was applied and fine grain industrial type of film was
used.   With this technique, highly satisfactory roentgenograms were obtained in nearly
every instance.   In the 16 carcinomas in their series, evidence of psammomatous calcification was obtained on roentgenograms in only three, but on specimen roentgenograms
this was demonstrated in 6 cases.   However, on histologic sections psammoma bodies
were actually found in 10 of them.   These results indicated that more than half of the
cancers did in fact contain psammoma bodies, but most of the instances had too few
psammoma bodies to be seen even on these special roentgenograms.   Thus, in spite of
the technical refinement, the discouraging results led them to conclude that there was
little to recommend its routine use in the evaluation of thyroid nodules.   Their opinion
was quite conservative, stating that "....This method of study may well be useful when
clinical findings strongly indicate that a nodule is malignant.   It may be further applied
as a supplement to routine roentgen examination in which deposits of calcification are
considered suspicious."

OUTLINE OF AUTHORS' INVESTIGATION

From 1968 through 1970, a research group was organized with the goal of "Development of Methods for the Early Diagnosis of the Breast and Thyroid Cancers" supported
by a research grant from the Ministry of Welfare of Japan.   One of the authors (Y. F.)
was chosen as a member, as he had been working in the surgical area of thyroidology
since 1955.   Dr. M. FUJIMORI, Professor of General Surgery, University of Gumma and the
chief of the research group, majored in both areas of breast and thyroid cancer, and
provided the opportunity for cooperation and exchange of knowledge between the two
subgroups.   The main subjects discussed in the diagnostic methods in breast carcinoma were palpation, mammography and ultrasound scanning, and the subjects in
thyroid carcinoma were palpation, scintiscanning and ultrasound scanning.   Therefore
it was quite natural that the application of soft tissue roentgenographic technique that
proved so useful in the diagnois of the breast cancer was also considered worth trying
in the field of thyroid cancer.   Then, the other author of this monograph (M. A.) was
asked to join the group, who had been using soft tissue radiography as a diagnostic aid for
lesions of the breast and had reviewed mammographs of more than 1,000 histologically
proven cases.

The first problem considered was the applicability of soft tissue roentgenography in the
demonstration of thyroid lesions.   The reason for successful mammography lies in the
anatomical position, shape and composition of the breast.   The breast contains a fairly
large amount of radiolucent adipose tissue, whereas the thyroid tissue is rich in epithelial
cells and colloid, and in addition the gland is surrounded by muscles.   Therefore, it was
thought to be extremely difficult to demonstrate thyroid tumors as a mass with increased

density enough for identification on roentgenograms of the neck. With these unfavorable factors in mind, we had one hope that calcifications a having higher radiological density might be shown on roentgenograms of the neck, the incidence of which is much higher than in the breast carcinomas. The pattern of calcification that has diagnostic significance is a psammomatous one and histologically psammoma bodies are shown to be contained in more than half of the thyroid cancers.

Thus, from the start of our study, the aim of soft tissue roentgenography of the thyroid gland was focused mainly on the demonstration of psammomatous calcification, and not on the demonstration of the tumor shadows and other auxiliary findings such as increased vascularity and thickening of adjacent structure as in mammography.

At the intermediate report meeting held in December, 1969, WATANABE and his collaborators, who were members of the research group, reported that they obtained roentgenographic evidence of calcific deposits including both coarse and psammomatous patterns in 51 of 78 thyroid cancers, or 65.4%, and in 48 of 185 benign adenomas, or 25.9%. This exceedingly high incidence of calcification stimulated us strongly. Our actual study began immediately after the meeting.

As the first step of our study, routine roentgenograms of the neck were retrospectively reviewed, which had been obtained prior to December, 1969. One hundred consecutive patients with histologically proven carcinomas and 100 patients with proven benign nodules were chosen as the material. In conjunction with the above study, roentgenograms of paraffin block specimens were obtained using soft tissue x-ray technique and findings were correlated with the histological appearances. Routine neck x-ray films were taken with the following technical factors: 150 cm, 78 kVp, 200 mA, 0.16 sec., for the antero-posterior view and 150 cm, 72 kVp, 200 mA, 0.12 sec. for the lateral view. For both projections, medical films were used with a type FS intensifying screen and Bucky 5: 1. In our clinic, only displacement or compression of the trachea had been evaluated on those roentgenograms and no special attention had been paid to the presence of calcifications.

Table 1 Retrospective Study on Calcifications in 100 Consecutive Patients with Proven Thyroid Cancers and 100 Consecutive Patients with Proven Benign Nodules.

Pathological classification	Preoperative roentgenograms of the neck		Specimen roentgenograms and histologic sections	
	No. available for review	Calcification present	No. available for examination	Calcification present
Thyroid cancer	75	32 (42.7%)	100	78 (78.0%)
Benign thyroid nodule	72	11 (15.3%)	98	46 (47.0%)

Seventy-five patients in cancer group and 72 patients in benign nodule group had lateral views of the neck available for review. As shown in Table 1, calcifications were found histologically in 78 cases of a total of 100 cancer patients, but found in only 32 out of 75 roentgenograms of the neck, or 42.7%. In the group of benign thyroid nodules, calcifications were found histologically in 47% and roentgenologically in 15.3%. The roentgenographic appearances observed were classified into 10 patterns. As shown in Table 2, the punctate, the nebular and the coarse irregular pattern were frequently seen in the cancers, and the curvilinear, coarse amorphous deposit and circular type were more often seen in the benign nodules. But it was true that these roentgenograms lacked detail and strict classification of patterns of calcification was rather difficult. No specific pattern was

Table 2 Patterns of Calcification Observed on Routine Neck Roentgenograms.

		Pathological classification	
		Thyroid cancer	Benign thyroid nodule
Spiculated		1	0
Linear		3	1
Grossly punctate		1	2
Punctate		11	1
Nebular		6	2
Coarse irregular		4	0
Coarse homogeneous		3	1
Circular		3	2
Coarse amorphous		0	1
Curvilinear		0	1
Total		32	11

found which was pathognomonic of cancer. It is because only psammoma bodies in sufficient numbers and of conglomerated form were shown on the roentgenograms and their shadows were of so poorly delineated that they were easily confused with the coarse irregular calcific deposits. Psammoma bodies of insufficient numbers were almost completely excluded from roentgenologic demonstration. This fact is apparent in Table 3, which shows the results of correlative study of the roentgenographic appearance with the histologic findings in the cancer group. Of 22 carcinomas that had the histological evidence of both coarse and psammomatous calcifications, 18 showed calcific shadows of a variety of configulations, mostly coarse patterns. Of 15 carcinomas that had only coarse calcific deposits on histologic sections, 10 showed the deposits on the neck x-ray. Of prime importance was the observation that in the 25 instances in which cancers had only psammoma bodies on histologic sections, only two showed calcific shadows on roentgenograms of the neck, the remainder showing no calcification. Thus, the result of the first step of our study clearly indicated that the standard roentgenograms of the neck were noncontributory as far as the demonstration of psammoma bodies was concerned.

Table 3 Calcification in Thyroid Cancers——Correlative study of neck roentgenograms with surgical specimen roentgenograms and histologic sections.

Calcification on neck roentgenograms	No. of patients	Calcification identified on specimen roentgenograms and histologic sections			
		None	Coarse calcification alone	Psammoma bodies alone	Combined
Present	32	2	10	2	18
Absent	43	11	5	23	4
Total	75	13	15	25	22

The results of the roentgenographic study of the paraffin-block specimens and their correlation with the histologic appearances will be described in detail in the following chapter.

We recognized the need for technical improvement in roentgenography and started the second step of the study, an *in vitro* phantom experiment.

Initially the tests were performed the lateral projection, and trial of every available technique produced roentgenograms of insufficient detail and contrast. Psammoma bodies were only poorly shown on the films in this projection. After discussion with one of our colleagues, Dr. E. TAKENAKA, we arrived at two simple, but very important principles, *i.e.*, firstly to minimize the inclusion of soft tissue mass by using a tangential projection, and secondly to collimate the x-ray beam with the use of a narrow cylinder cone, although the field of observation is significantly reduced. At the time of these studies, we already had reviewed most of the literature concerning the use of soft tissue roentgenography in the diagnosis of thyroid cancer, but we apparently went through them rather superficially. After having attained satisfactory roentgenograms in the phantom experiment, we reread those papers and realized their deep consideration of the technical details for the first time.

The authors proceeded to the clinical application of the method which had proven to be satisfactory in a water phantom study. A surgeon (Y. F.) and a radiologist (M. A.) worked together and in each case the results of preoperative physical examination, neck x-ray, macroscopic finding at operation, specimen roentgenogram and histologic examination were carefully checked and all the results were correlated. We were quite fortunate in that we periodically encountered patients with thyroid lesions which were considered benign on the routine physical and laboratory examinations, but roentgenograms of the neck definitely showed psammomatous calcifications and thus the preoperative diagnosis of cancer was made. Such experiences constantly encouraged us in continuing our work.

Chapter II

Roentgenographic-Histologic Patterns of Calcification in Thyroid Nodules

The calcifications occurring in thyroid nodules present a great variety of forms on roentgenograms of the neck. Thus far several investigators have attempted to formulate the criteria by which differentiation of benign and malignant nodules may be roentgenologically possible. It has been generally agreed that, when calcium deposits in the thyroid nodules are grossly classified into two types, "psammomatous" and "coarse", the former has diagnostic value because of its occurrence almost exclusively in cases of thyroid carcinoma, whereas the latter bears no relationship to the histologic diagnosis.

In order to confirm the above criteria, we analized various patterns of thyroid calcification on specimen roentgenograms and the findings were correlated with the histologic appearance.

The purpose of this study lies in the understanding of the variety of forms and patterns of calcification which had developed in pathologic processes of the thyroid gland. How to visualize psammoma bodies on the roentgenogram of the neck is another problem and will be discussed in the following chapter.

MATERIALS AND METHODS

Roentgenographic and histologic examinations were carried out retrospectively on surgically ermoved specimens of 100 consecutive patients with malignant thyroid neoplasms and 98 with benign nodules including adenoma and adenomatous goiter. The operations were performed at the Second Department of Surgery, University of Tokyo, prior to December, 1969. Fine-grain industrial film (Sakura X-Ray Film, Type MR) and low kilo-voltage were used to obtain the maximum detail in specimen roentgenograms.

Initially roentgenograms were made on both the paraffin blocks of the surgically removed specimens and the remnants of the fixed specimens. After examining 39 cases of malignant tumors and 41 of benign nodules, we discontinued making roentgenograms of the remnants, because it became apparent that almost all the important portions of each specimen had been made into paraffin blocks and therefore the roentgenograms of the blocks provided enough material for analysis. In addition, roentgenograms of the remnant specimens were in general difficult to interpret because of their irregularity in shape and thickness and gave very little additional information.

The number of paraffin blocks in each case was one to 17, averaging 6.7 in malignant tumors and 3.7 in benign nodules. Although specimens which had readily recognizable gross calcifications and had been demineralized before processing to the paraffin blocks did not show calcific deposits on the roentgenograms, they were treated as having coarse calcification and the calcified areas were usually identified on the microscopic sections by their blue staining with hematoxylin. The histology sections stained by hematoxylin and eosin were examined in all cases, and later in 24 selected sections representing all of the characteristic patterns of calcification silver nitrate staining by von KÓSSA's method was used.

INCIDENCE OF CALCIFICATIONS IN MALIGNANT
AND BENIGN THYROID NODULES

Calcium deposits observed on specimen roentgenograms were initially divided into two types; psammomatous and coarse. When roentgenograms of excised specimens were carefully checked and the findings were correlated with the histologic features, both types of thyroid calcification were detected in an unexpectedly high percentage of cases. The incidences in the benign and the malignant nodules are shown in Table 4.

Table 4 Incidence of Calcification Seen on Roentgenograms of Thyroidectomy Specimens.

Histologic diagnosis	Total No. of cases	No. of cases with calcification*			Calcification positive rate	
		Ps^+ Co^+	Ps^+ Co^-	Ps^- Co^+	Psammo-matous %	Coarse %
Malignant neoplasms						
Papillary carcinoma	79	17	31	14	60.7	39.3
Follicular carcinoma	12	4	1	4	41.7	66.7
Medullary carcinoma	5	1	4	0	100.0	20.0
Papillary carcinoma associated with anaplastic carcinoma	2	1	0	1	50.0	100.0
Malignant lymphoma	2	0	0	0	0	0
Total	100	23	36	19	59.0	42.0
Benign nodules						
Adenoma	72	0	1	26	1.4	36.1
Adenomatous goiter	26	0	1	16	3.8	61.6
Total	98	0	2	42	2.0	42.8

*Ps: Psammomatous calcification.
 Co: Coarse calcification.
 "Ps+, Co+" indicates cases which had both psammomatous and coarse calcifications.

Psammomatous calcification was seen in 59 of 100 malignant tumors, whereas it was present in only two of 98 benign nodules.

As to the distribution by histologic type, psammomatous calcification was common in the papillary and the medullary carcinomas and less frequently seen in the follicular carcinoma. As will be shown in the following paragraph, however, of these psammomatous calcification positive cancers, four cases of papillary carcinoma and two cases of follicular carcinoma had in fact no true psammoma bodies, but had minute calcific deposits in the fibrous stroma within the neoplasms, and most of the psammomatous shadows observed on specimen roentgenograms of four medullary carcinomas were revealed histologically to be due to calcium deposits within the amyloid.

The incidence of coarse calcification in malignant tumors was the same as in benign nodules in our series.

ROENTGENOGRAPHIC AND HISTOLOGIC APPEARANCE OF THYROID CALCIFICATION

1. Roentgenographic Psammomatous Calcification

Although most of the calcium deposits showing a psammomatous pattern on roentgenograms were proved histologically to be true psammoma bodies, there were some other calcific deposits which presented a similar pattern.

a. Psammoma Bodies

As for the development and distribution of psammoma bodies, several patterns were observed. The patterns commonly seen are as follows;

Type 1: Evenly scattered psammoma bodies without forming conglomerates.
Type 2: Psammoma bodies associated with larger, round calcific bodies.
Type 3: Aggregates of psammoma bodies that are histologically found in the tips of papillary stalks projected in the cystic areas of papillary cancers.
Type 4: Diffuse distribution of psammoma bodies throughout the thyroid tissue.

The most typical appearance of psammoma bodies is represented by type 1 and shown in case 1 (Fig. 1-a, b and c). The roentgenologic appearance is like very small grains of sand scattered about. Most of the calcific deposits on the specimen roentgenogram (Fig. 1-a) represent individual psammoma bodies, which are usually 20 to 70 μ in diameter. Their roentgenologic density is too low to be seen on the ordinary roentgenogram of the neck. They tend to be distributed heavily at the periphery of the tumor. Psammoma bodies of this type are most commonly seen in the papillary carcinoma with histologic evidence of active infiltrative proliferation. The bodies also appear in the clusters of cancer cells which have invaded into lymphatic vessels in the adjacent thyroid tissue near the primary tumor.

The specimen roentgenogram of Case 2 (Fig. 2-a) shows an example of type 2 psammomatous calcification. It is characterized by a mixture of fine sand-like calcific grains and larger, round calcific bodies. Histologic sections showed that even the fine deposits seen in this case were made up of a clump of several psammoma bodies. The round, dense calcific deposits, with the size up to 1 mm in diameter, appeared to develop as a result of calcium deposition in degenerated cellular masses which were included within dense fibrosis. Because of an increase in density and size, psammomatous calcifications of this type are readily recognizable on the neck roentgenogram.

The next two cases (Case 3 and 4) show type 3 psammoma bodies. The bodies tend to appear in the tip of the papillary stalks. They usually take the form of a mixture of variably sized irregular aggregates and fine scattered grains. Case 4 demonstrates a far advanced stage of the process, in which the papillary stalk itself has undergone marked degenerative change within the cystic space. The psammoma bodies are numerous and conglomerated, so that they give denser and larger psammomatous shadows on the film. The papillary carcinomas that contain this type of psammoma bodies are usually not invasive and on physical examination occasionally simulate benign nodules.

Case 5 (Fig. 5-a, b and c) shows type 4 psammomatous calcification. The papillary carcinoma of this type is characterized by a remarkable extension of cancer cells into lymphatic channels in the thyroid tissue around the primary growth, the extension being often so intense that the whole thyroid may be involved. This type of carcinoma is usually seen in female patients younger than 25 years old and has an associated chronic thyroiditis.

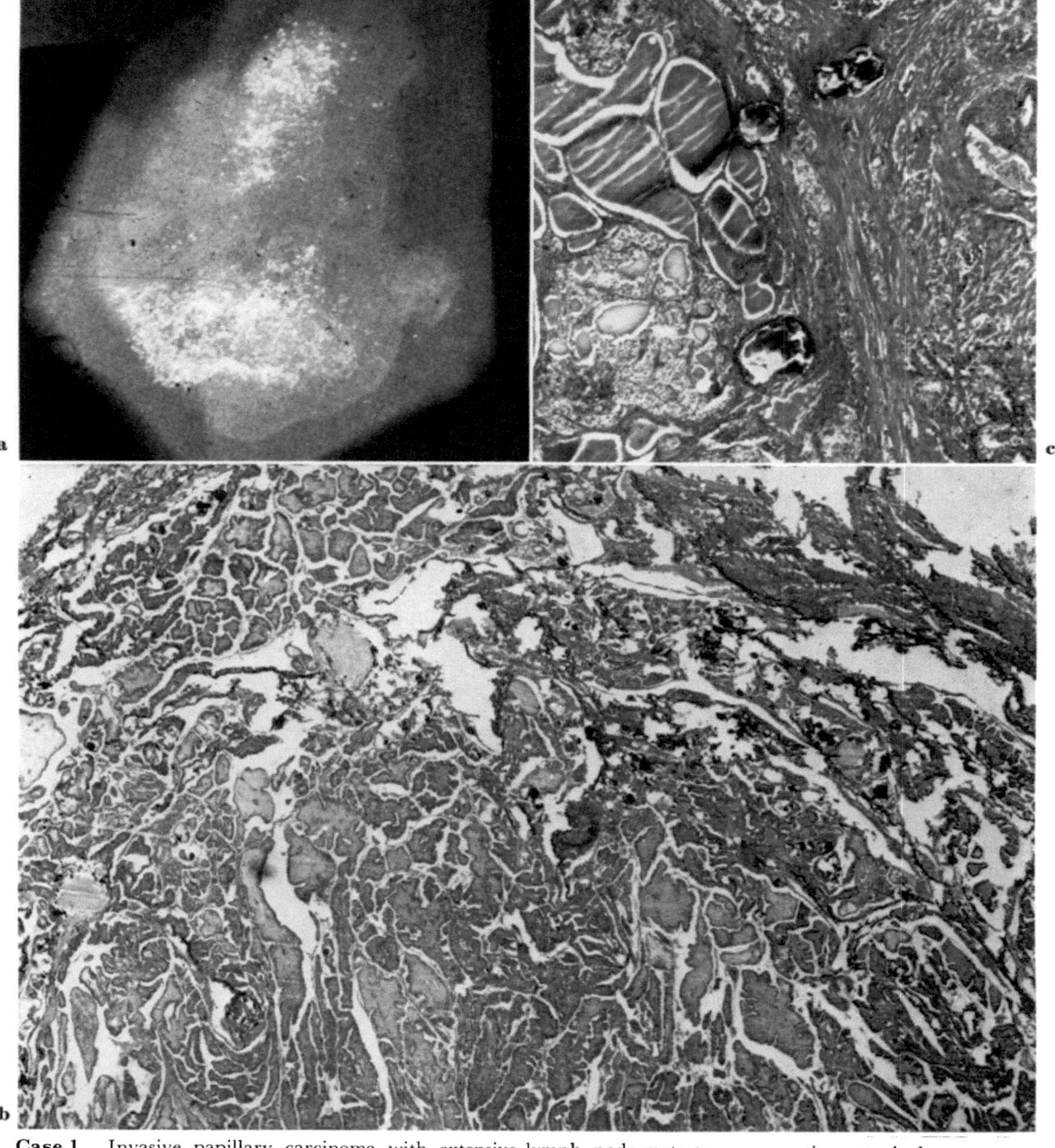

Case 1 Invasive papillary carcinoma with extensive lymph node metastases, presenting a typical psammomatous pattern of calcification (# 683543, N. H., 26 year-old male).

Fig. 1-a Roentgenogram of paraffin block specimen, showing a psammomatous pattern of calcification due to evenly scattered psammoma bodies (×2.5).

Fig. 1-b Low power photomicrograph of specimen, showing psammoma bodies appearing mostly at the periphery of the cancer (H & E, ×15).

Fig. 1-c High power photomicrograph of specimen. Psammoma bodies are basophilic, concentrically laminated, calcified structures, measuring 20 to 70 μ in diameter. The bodies appear in the interlobular fibrous tissue and block the lymphatic canals (H & E, ×50).

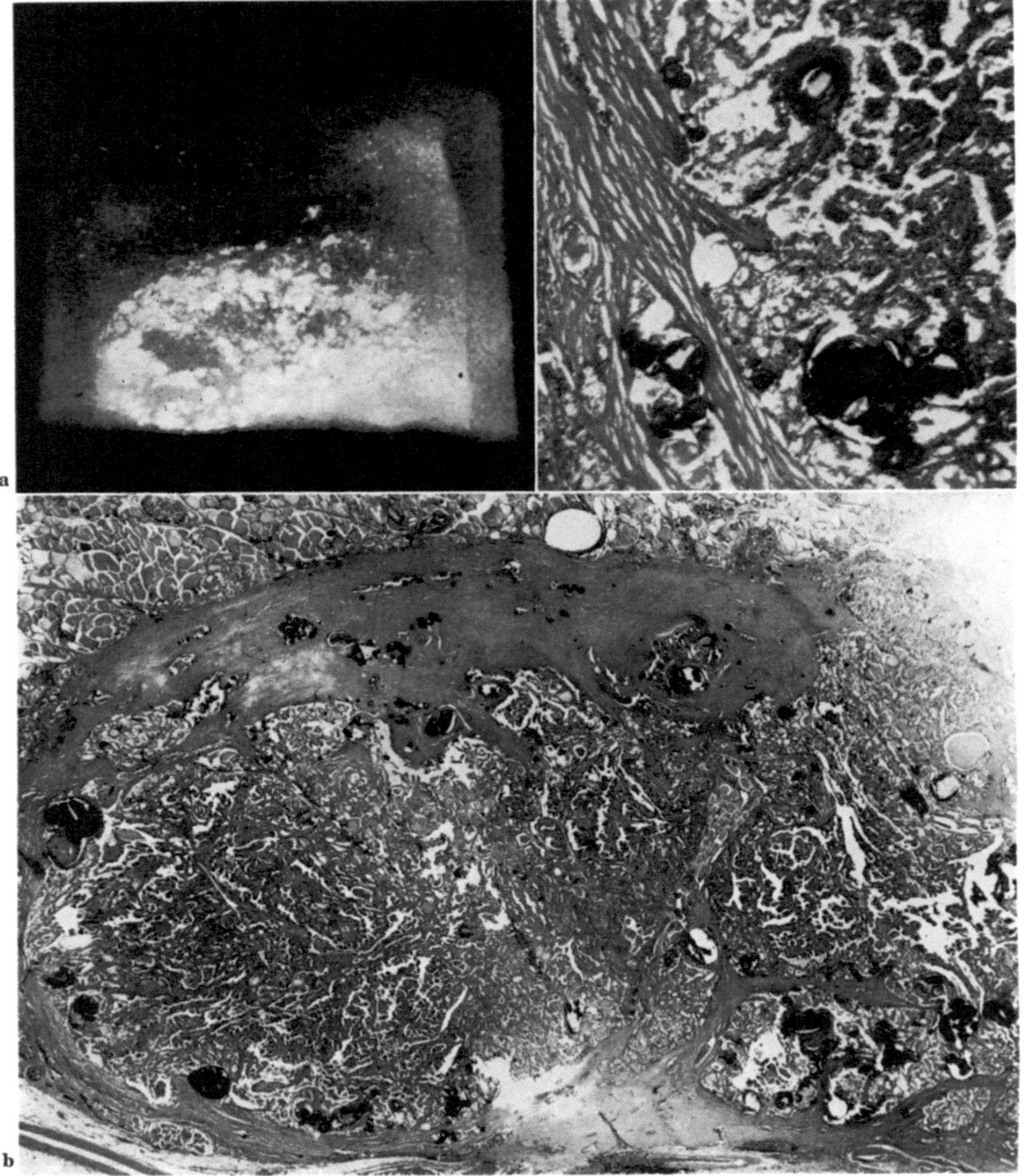

Case 2 Papillary carcinoma with extensive lymph node metastases, presenting a psammomatous pattern of calcification (No. 715607, M. U., 33 year-old female).

Fig. 2-a Roentgenogram of paraffin block specimen, showing typical psammomatous calcification associated with larger round calcific granules in the lower half of the paraffin block which is occupied by cancer. Also note the scattered psammomatous calcifications in the remnant thyroid in the upper half of the block ($\times 2.5$).

Fig. 2-b Low power photomicrograph of specimen. Calcified bodies and granules appeared predominantly within and around the tumor capsule (H & E, $\times 7$).

Fig. 2-c High power view of hisotlogic section (H & E, $\times 100$).

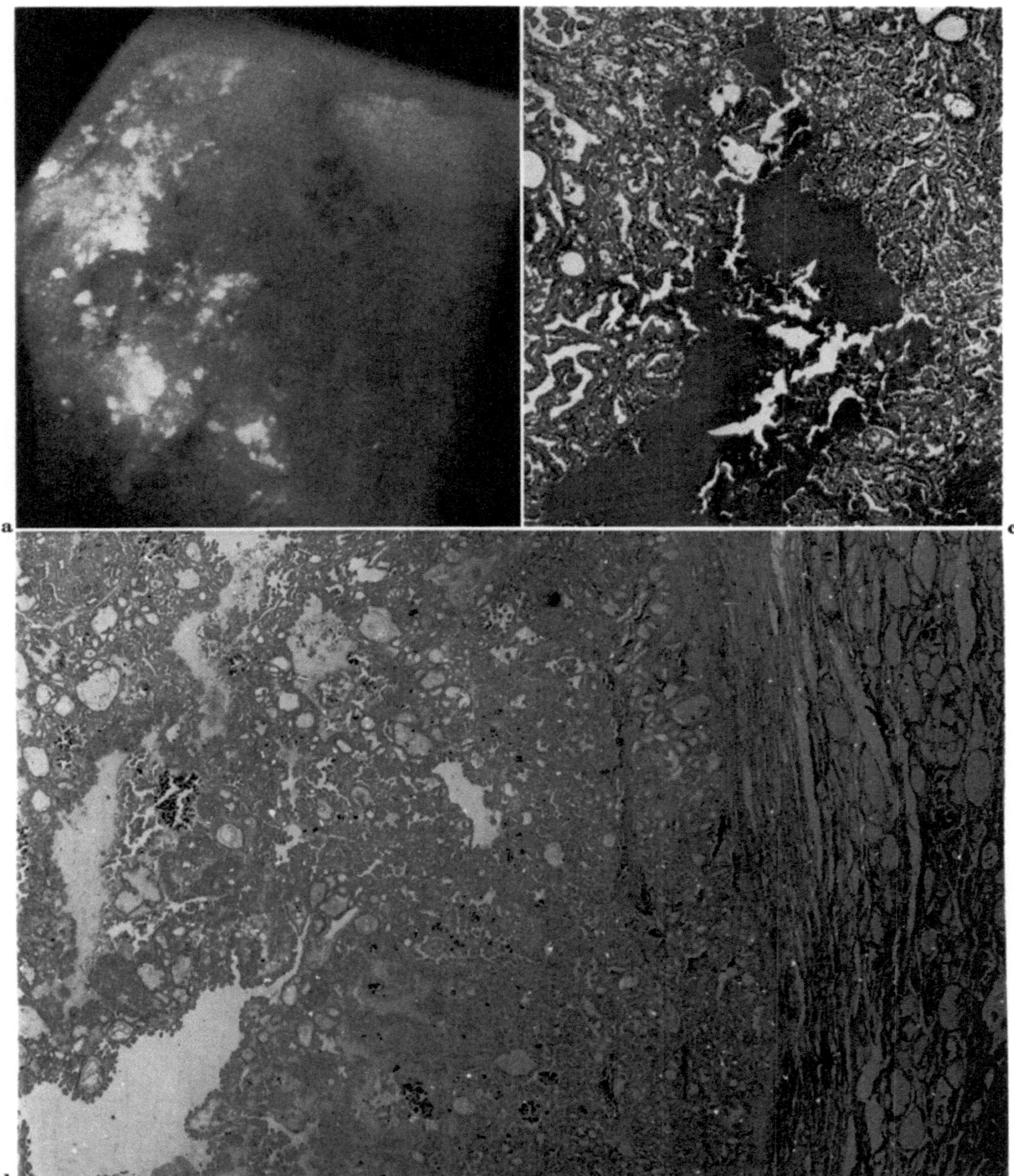

Case 3   Encapsulated papillary carcinoma without evidence of lymph node metasis, presenting aggregates of psammoma bodies at the tips of papillary proliferation (# 674499, A. H., 26 year-old male).

Fig. 3-a   Roentgenogram of the paraffin specimen, showing a mixture of scattered fine grains and variable sized, irregular aggregates ($\times 2.5$).

Fig. 3-b   Low power photomicrograph of specimen (Kóssa, $\times 10$).

Fig. 3-c   High power photomicrograph of specimen. Psammoma bodies tend to concentrate in aggregates in the tips of papillary stalks projected into the cystic areas of papillary cancer (Kóssa, $\times 50$).

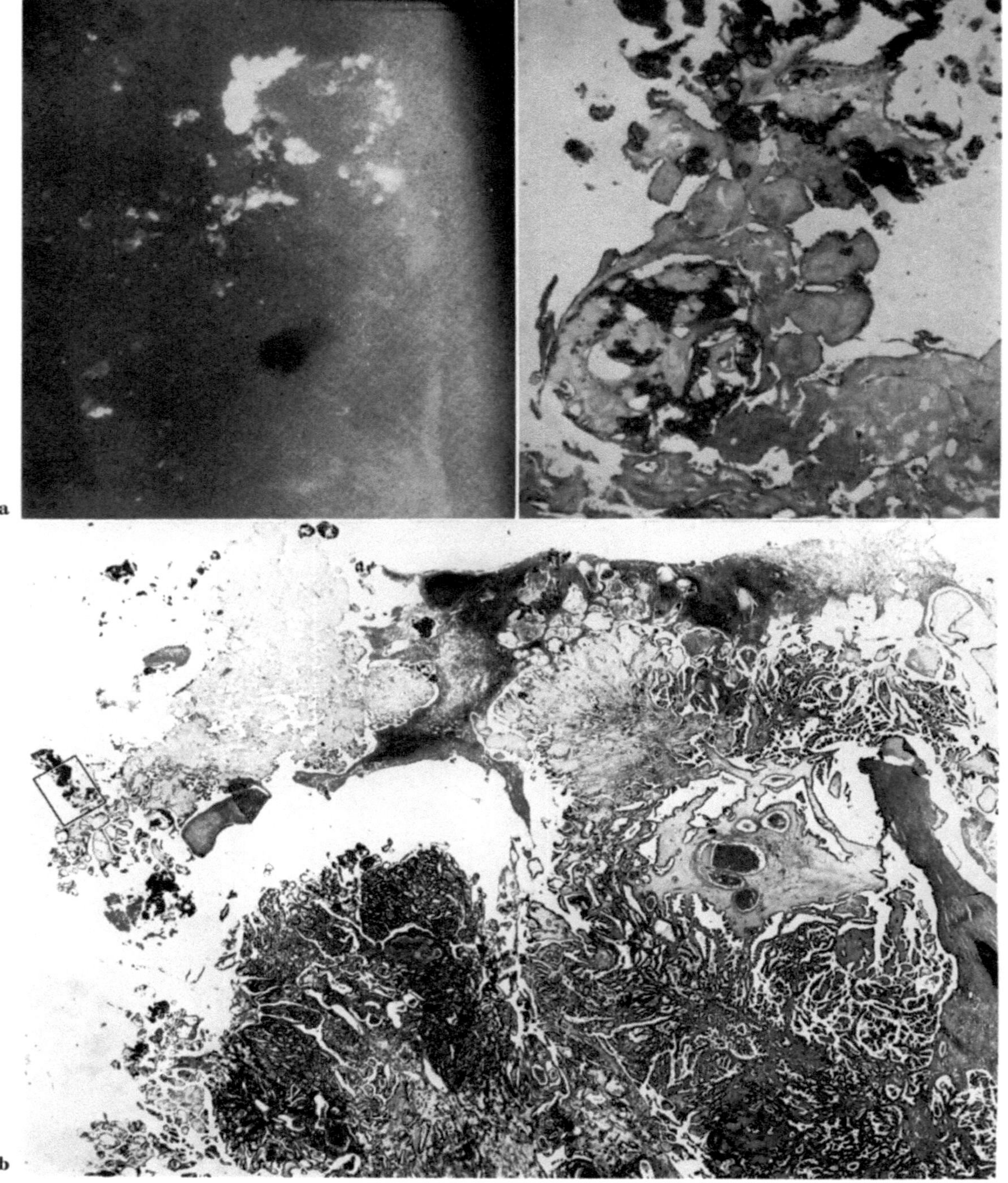

Case 4   Encapsulated papillary carcinoma with lymph node metastases, presenting psammoma bodies of conglomerated form (# 663743, M. T., 74 year-old male).

Fig. 4-a   Roentgenogram of the paraffin block specimen, showing amorphous dense calcification and shadows
of scattered and conglomerated psammoma bodies ($\times 2.5$).

Fig. 4-b   Low power photomicrograph of specimen, showing typical papillary proliferation.   In the left upper
and middle upper portions, the papillary carcinoma underwent degenerative change and psammoma bodies
appear in conglomerated form.   At the right corner, densely calcified fibrous band is observed (H & E, $\times 7$).

Fig. 4-c   High power view of an area of abundant psammoma bodies (H & E, $\times 50$).

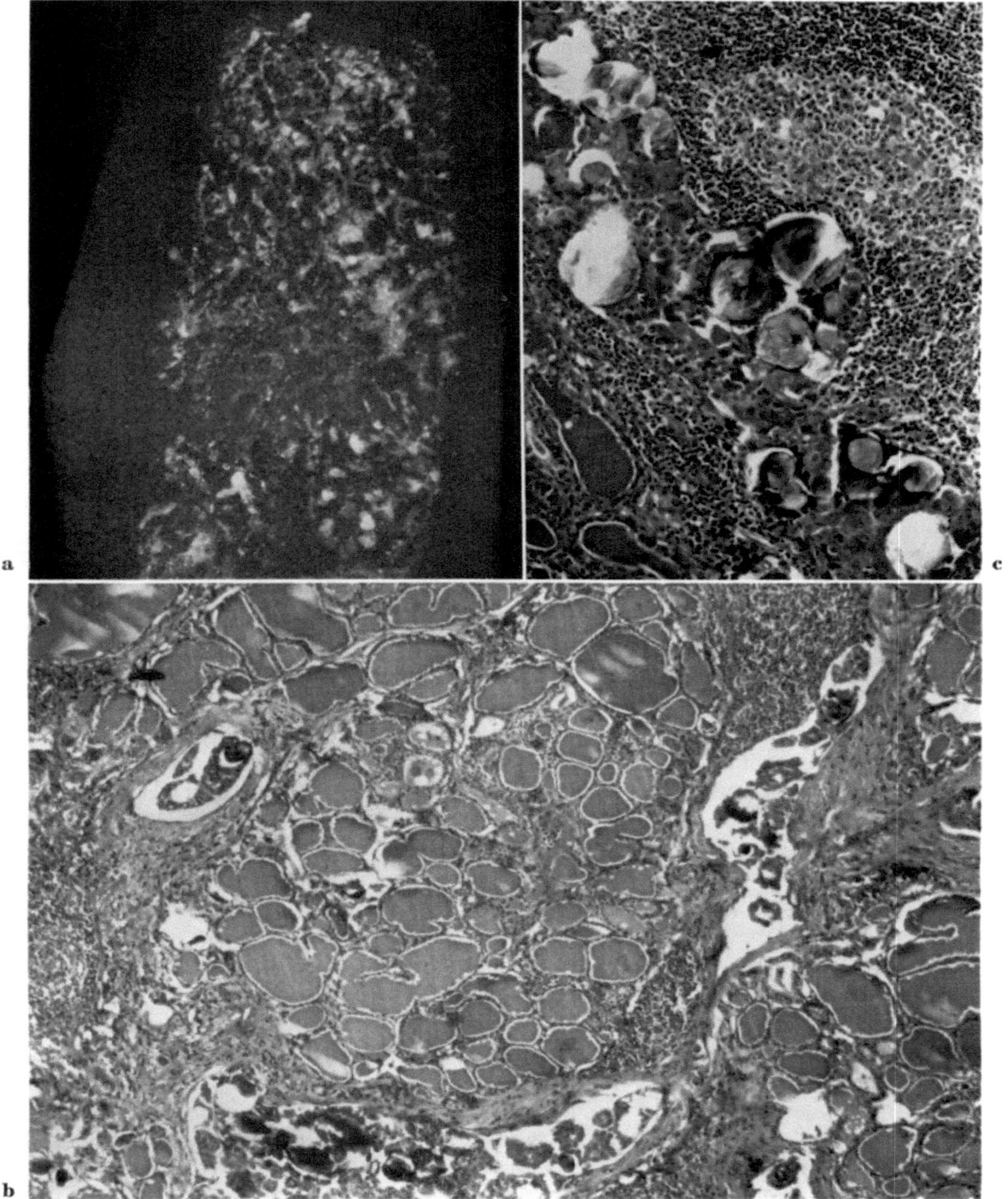

Case 5 Invasive papillary carcinoma showing diffusely distributed psammoma bodies throughout the thyroid tissue (♯ 43843, A. K., 19 year-old female).

Fig. 5-a Roentgenogram of paraffin block specimen, showing a network made up by very fine calcified grains. The roentgenographic appearance is similar to that of thyroid lymphography, which is obtained by direct *in vivo* injection of *Lipiodol Ultra-Fluid* into the thyroid tissue (×2.5).

Fig. 5-b Photomicrograph of specimen. This is a special type of papillary carcinoma characterized by remarkable intrathyroidal infiltration of cancer cells via lymphatic channels and association with chronic thyroiditis. Note many psammoma bodies developed in the infiltrating cancer cell clusters, and the appearance of lymph follicles as evidence of chronic thyroiditis (H & E, ×50).

Fig. 5-c High power view of the microscopic section, showing psammoma bodies having developed in intrathyroid extensions of papillary carcinoma via the interlobular lymphatic canals (H & E, ×100).

There are numerous psammoma bodies which have developed in cancer cell masses within lymphatic channels and hence thin strands of psammomatous shadows are seen throughout the thyroid parenchyma on the specimen roentgenogram.

b. Psammomatous Calcific Deposits Other Than Psammoma Bodies

Correlative roentgenographic and histologic study revealed that in a few cases calcific deposits other than psammoma bodies produced shadows very similar to those of psammoma bodies.

Among these, those seen mostly in papillary and the follicular carcinomas are minute calcific deposits in the fibrous stroma as shown in case 6 (Fig. 6-a and b).

Most of the fine deposits observed in medullary carcinoma were proved histologically to be calcific deposits in the amyloid (Fig. 7-a, b and c).

Psammomatous deposits were seen in one case of microfollicular adenoma and in one case of adenomatous goiter (Fig. 8-a and b).   Histologically it was difficult to confirm whether they were true psammoma bodies or calcific deposits at the site of degenerating epithelium.

2. Roentgenographically Coarse Calcification

Coarse calcification is seen in the fibrous stroma, septum and capsule of both benign and malignant nodules.   In the histologic sections stained with hematoxylin and eosin, only the areas where calcium is heavily deposited are stained dark blue and they correspond well with the form of calcification on the specimen roentgenogram, as seen in case 9 (papillary carcinoma, Fig. 9-a, b and c).   Calcification of low density is, however, actually present in the fibrous stroma around the dense deposits cited above and it only becomes apparent on sections stained by von Kóssa's method, as shown in case 13 (microfollicular adenoma, Fig. 13).

Roentgenographically coarse calcifications appear in various configurations, such as punctate, linear, curvilinear, irregular spicules or amorphous plaques of various sizes. Case 11 (papillary carcinoma) is one of the examples that contain various forms of coarse calcification.   In one area of the paraffin block specimen ossification is visible (Fig. 11-a and b).   Ossification was also observed in one benign nodule in our series.

In general, fibrosis and its calcification tend to be formed in an irregular fashion in the carcinomas as shown in case 9 and 11, and in a rather smooth configuration in the benign nodules as seen in case 12.   There are, however, exceptional cases such as seen in case 10 (carcinoma) and case 13 (adenoma).   Thus the configuration of calcification is not a reliable indication of the nature of the nodule, so far as the coarse calcification is concerned.

An extremely dense, amorphous type of calcification, occupying almost the whole area of the nodule, was seen in four cases; one was a well encapsulated papillary carcinoma with minimal capsular invasion, one was a Langhans' "wuchernde Struma" which had a rapidly growing, non-calcified small nodule protruded from the deeply seated, heavily calcified tumor mass (Cass 14, Fig. 14-a, b and c), one was a colloid adenoma and one was a benign nodule in which no viable tissue remained.

All the coarse calcifications described above are roentgenographically dense.   The fleece-like pattern seen in two adenomas was of low density.   Histological examination revealed that these particular calcific deposits were present along the sinusoidal vascular beds in the tumor parenchyma (Case 15, Fig. 15-b and c).

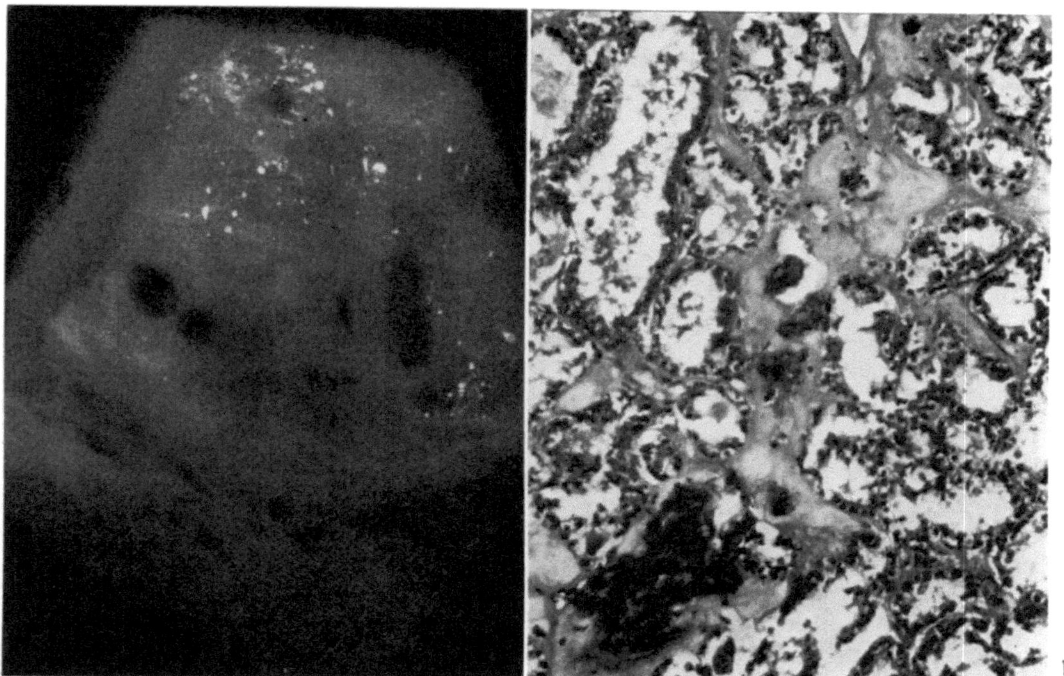

Case 6   Encapsulated papillary carcinoma without lymph node metastasis, presenting psammoma bodies mixed with minute calcific deposits in fibrous stroma (# 682027, Y. K., 59 year-old male).

Fig. 6-a   Roentgenogram of paraffin block specimen, showing irregular distribution of various size sand-like calcific shadows (×2.5).

Fig. 6-b   Photomicrograph of specimen, showing minute calcific deposits in the fibrous stroma of the cancer (H & E, ×120).

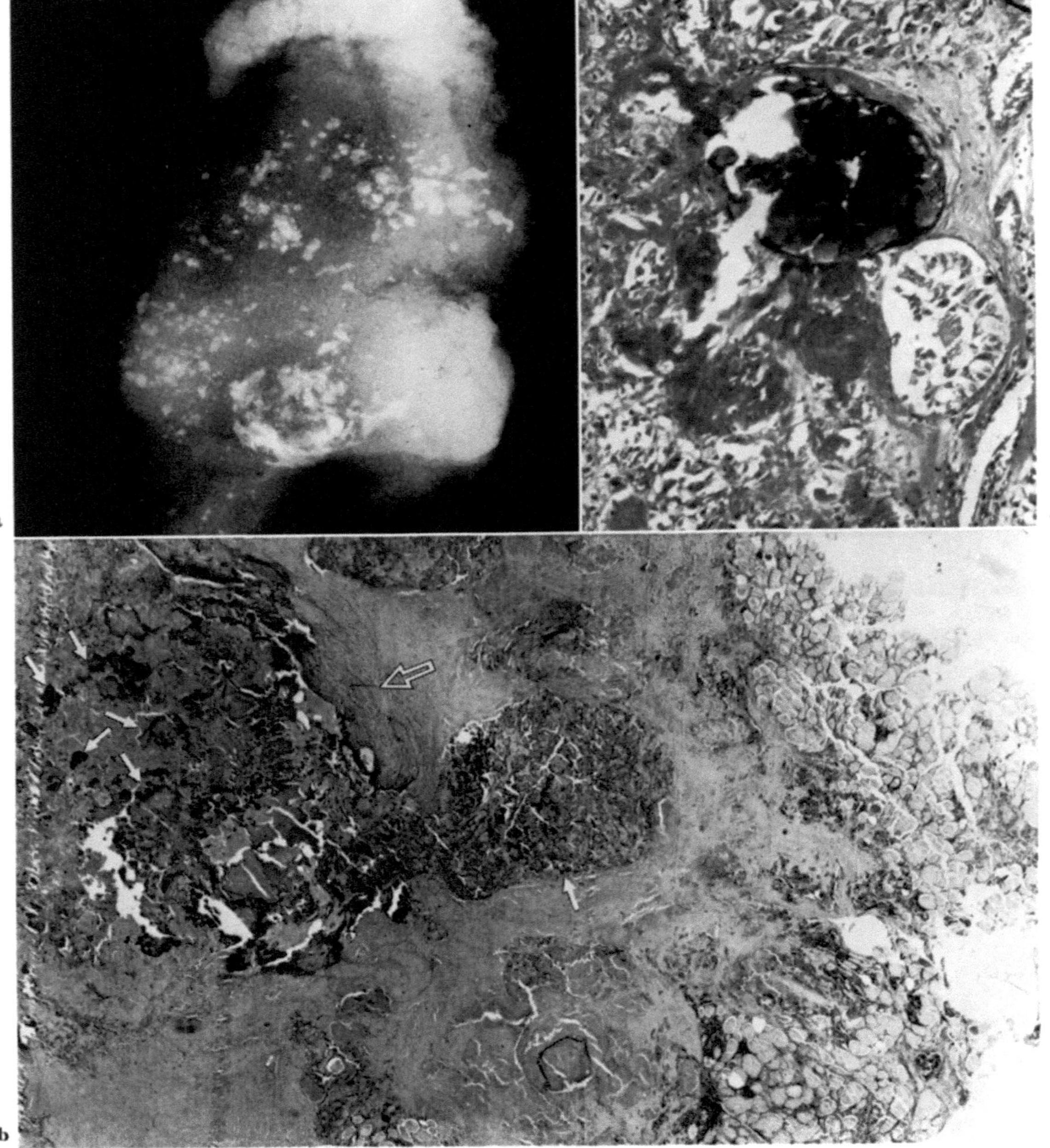

Case 7 Medullary carcinoma of the thyroid with remarkable lymph node metastases, showing psammoma-like calcific deposits (# 671551, K. A., 42 year-old female).

Fig. 7-a Roentgenogram of paraffin block specimen, showing scattered psammoma-like calcifications and coarse amorphous deposits below (×2.5).

Fig. 7-b Low power photomicrograph of specimen, showing a medullary carcinoma with abundant amyloid deposition and fibrosis. There are minute calcified granules in the areas of amyloid deposition (small arrows) and dense calcifications in the fibrosis (large arrow) (H & E, ×7).

Fig. 7-c High power view of specimen. A fairly large calcified granule appeared among the amyloid deposition (H & E, ×120).

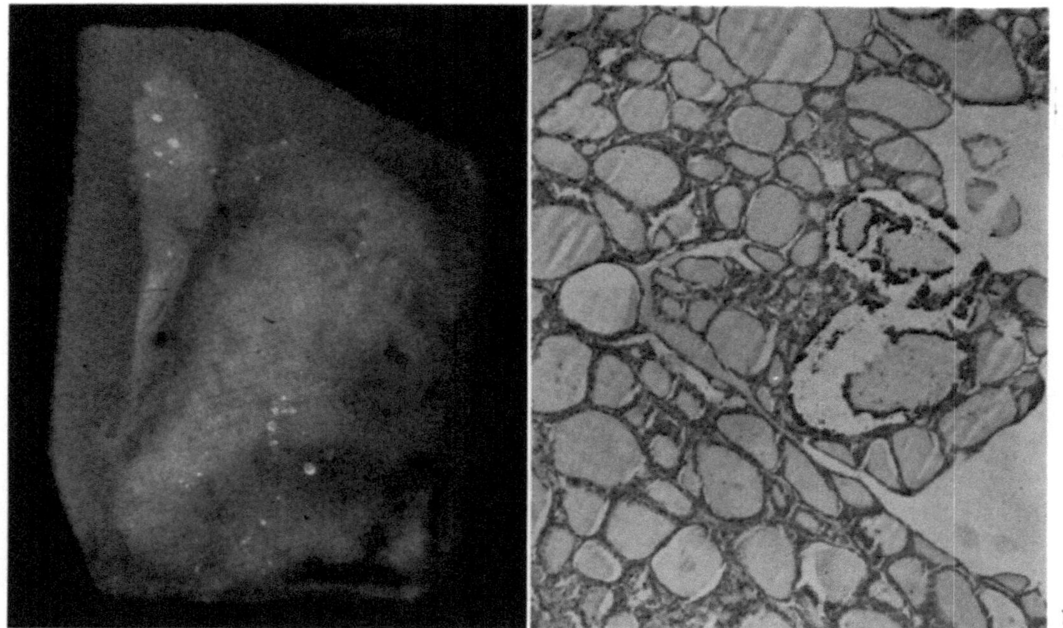

Case 8 Adenomatous goiter showing psammomatous calcification (# 673007, S. T., 53 year-old female).

Fig. 8-a Roentgenogram of paraffin block specimen, showing psammomatous calcification (×2.5).

Fig. 8-b Photomicrograph of specimen showing psammoma-like deposit of calcium (Kóssa, ×50).

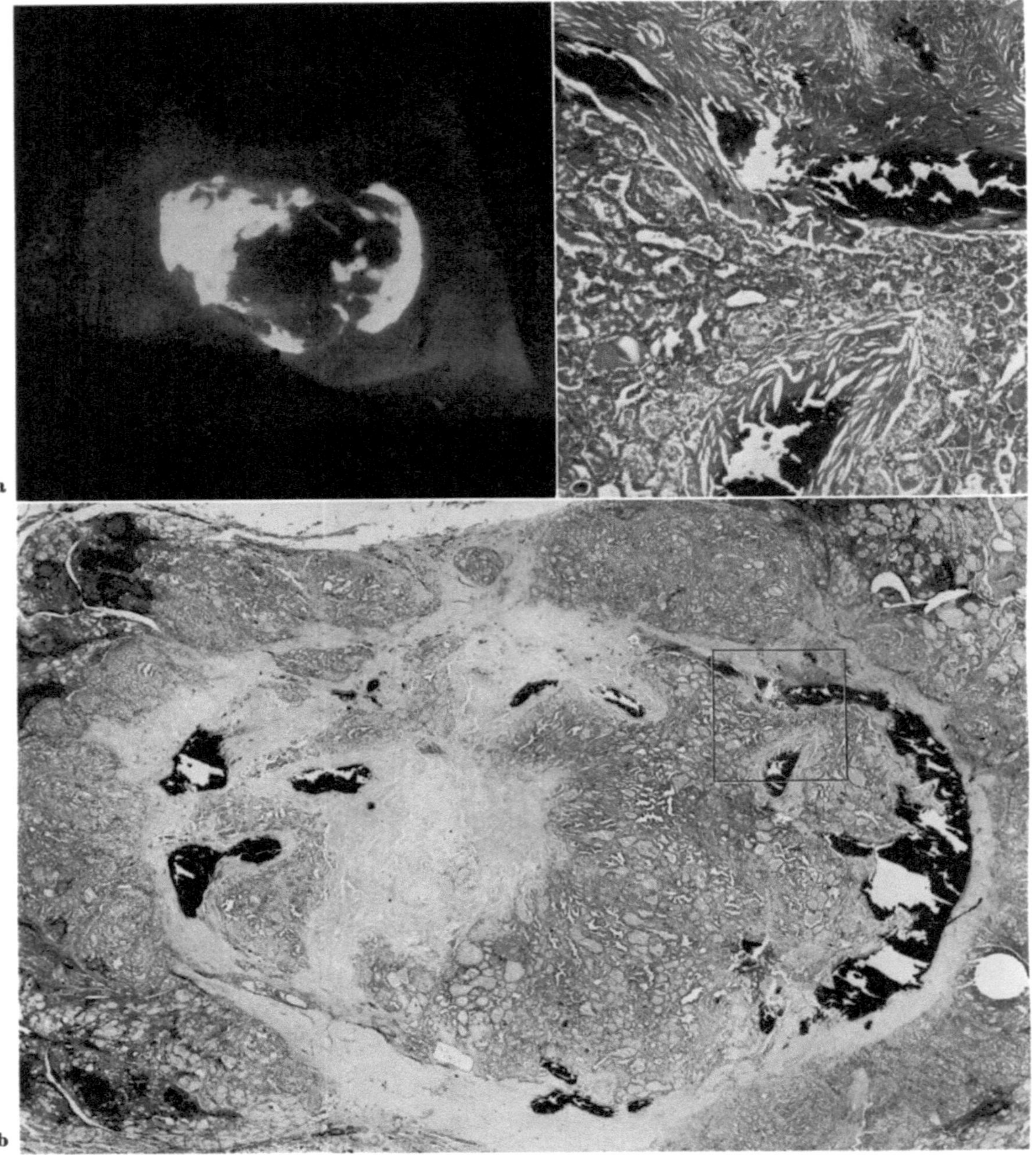

Case 9   Papillary carcinoma presenting coarse calcification in the fibrous capsule (# 686596, A. H., 26 year-old female).

Fig. 9-a   Roentgenogram of paraffin block specimen ($\times 2.5$).

Fig. 9-b   Low power photomicrograph of specimen.   Cancer tissue proliferates outside the calcified capsule and the uninvolved thyroid tissue is affected by chronic thyroiditis.   Roentgenographic appearance of calcification correlates quite well with histologic appearance. (H & E, $\times 10$).

Fig. 9-c   High power view of the tumor capsule (H & E, $\times 70$).

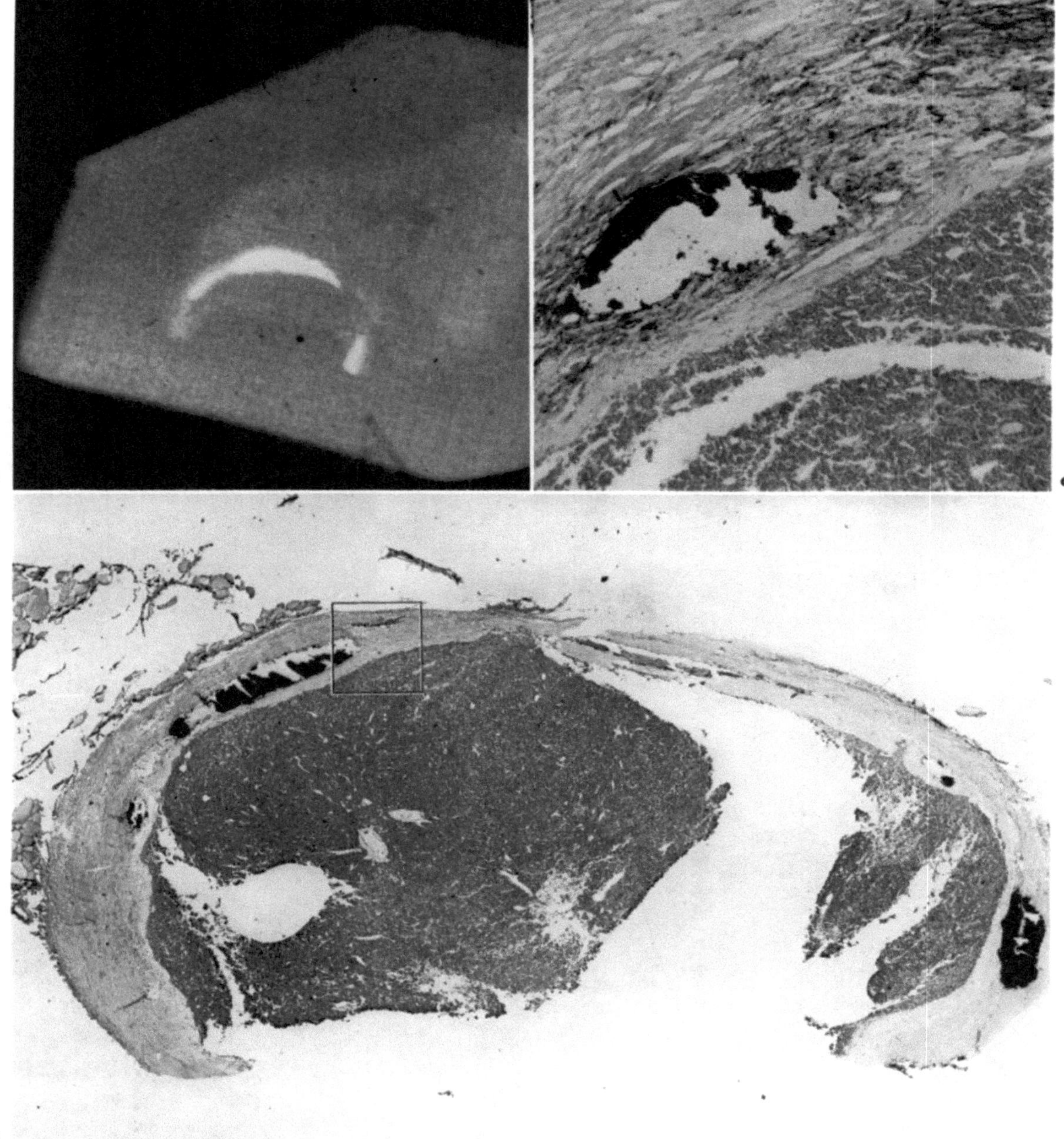

Case 10   Encapsulated follicular carcinoma presenting round coarse calcification (# 692751, K. S., 42 year-old female having a metastatic lesion in the pelvis).

Fig. 10-a   Roentgenogram of paraffin block specimen, showing a curvilinear calcification in the tumor capsule ($\times 2.5$).

Fig. 10-b   Low power photomicrograph of specimen, showing a follicular carcinoma 1 cm in diameter.   Note the densely calcified capsule (H & E, $\times 10$).

Fig. 10-c   High power view of the tumor capsule.   Calcification of low degree is demonstrated only by von Kóssa's staining, but unable to be demonstrated on the roentgenogram (Kóssa, $\times 50$).

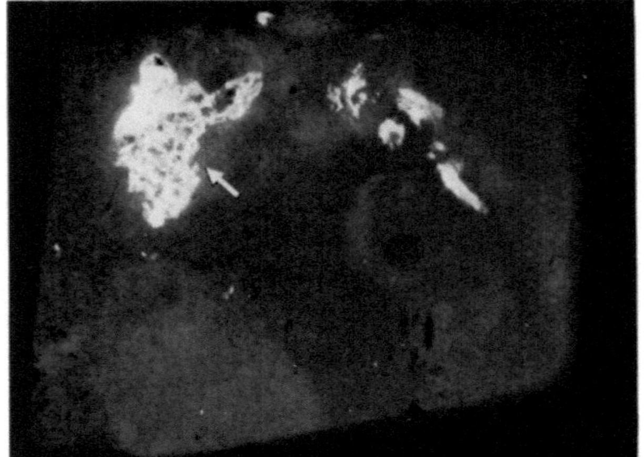

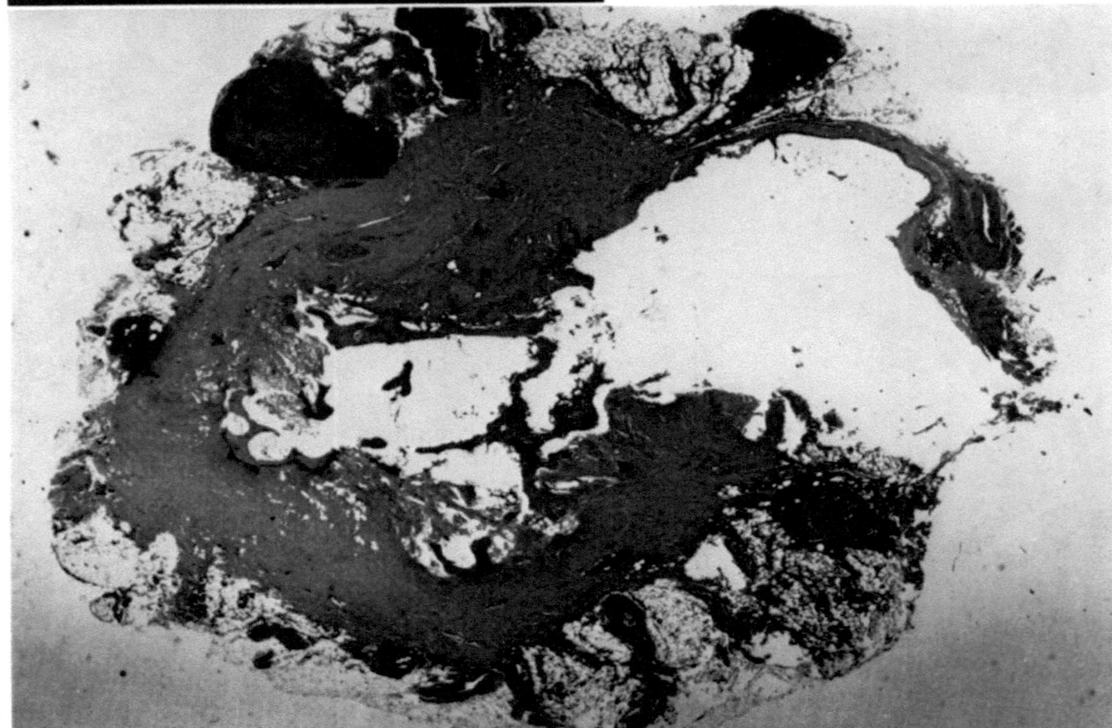

Case 11 Invasive papillary carcinoma showing coarse calcifications with variety of configurations. This case was first noticed due to recurrent laryngeal nerve palsy. There was no palpable nodule in the neck, but neck x-rays revealed compression of the trachea which suggested the presence of thyroid cancer (♯ 671176, M. T., 53 year-old female).

Fig. 11-a Roentgenogram of paraffin block specimen. The calcified network (arrow) represents ossification in the area of fibrosis in the cancer (×2.5).

Fig. 11-b Photomicrograph of the area of ossification (H & E, ×50).

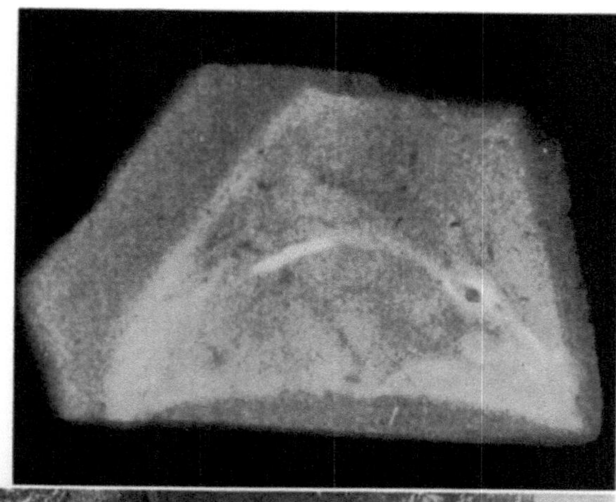

Case 12   Microfollicular adenoma showing coarse calcification in the fibrous trabecula (# 675955, K. N., 45 year-old female).

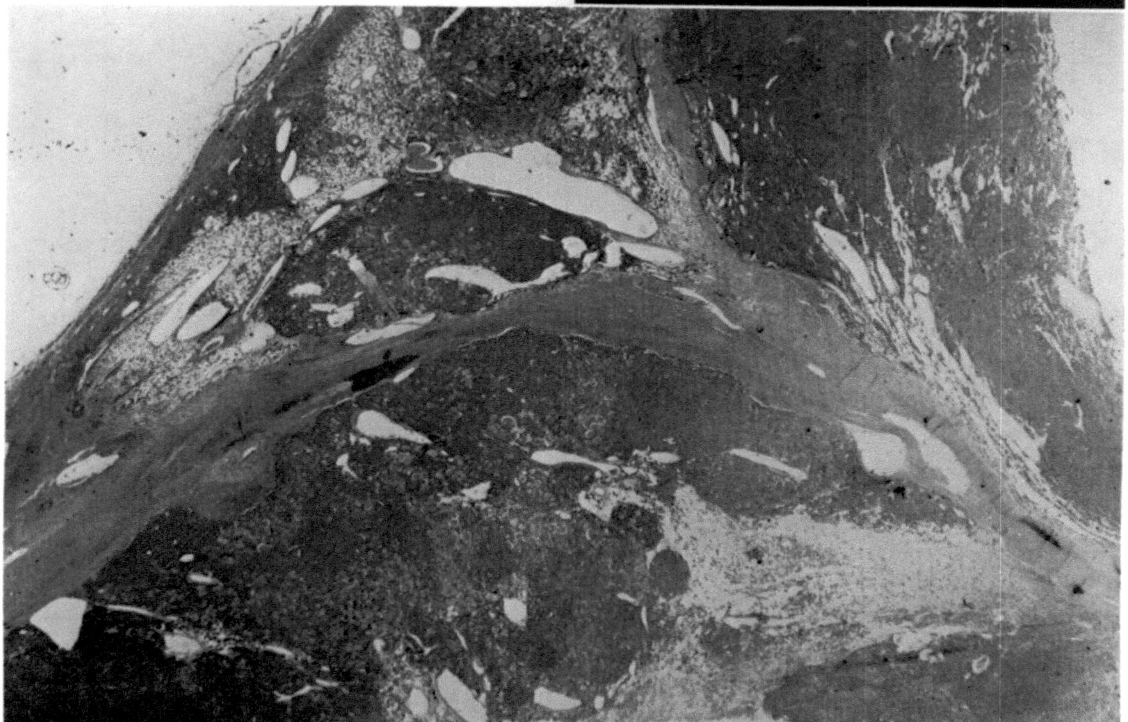

Fig. 12-a   Roentgenogram of paraffin block specimen (× 2.5).

Fig. 12-b   Photomicrograph of specimen (H & E, × 10).

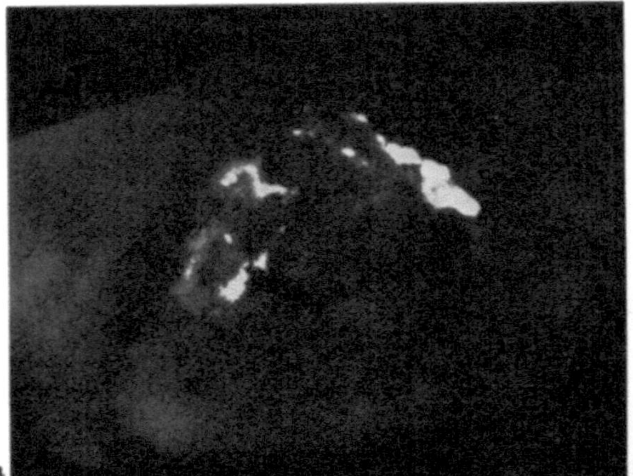

Case 13   Follicular adenoma showing coarse amorphous calcification in the capsule (# 663039, T. G., 47 year-old male).

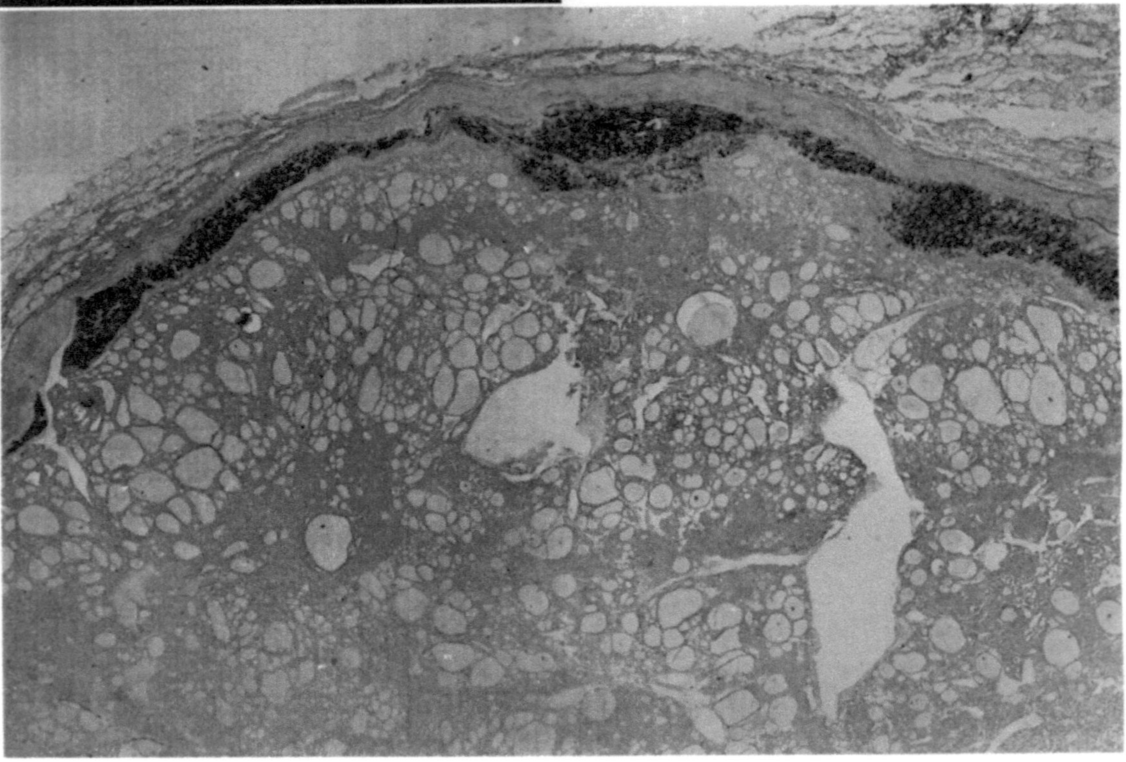

Fig. 13-a   Roentgenogram of paraffin block specimen (×2.5).

Fig. 13-b   Low power photomicrograph of specimen showing the calcified fibrous capsule (Kóssa, ×10).

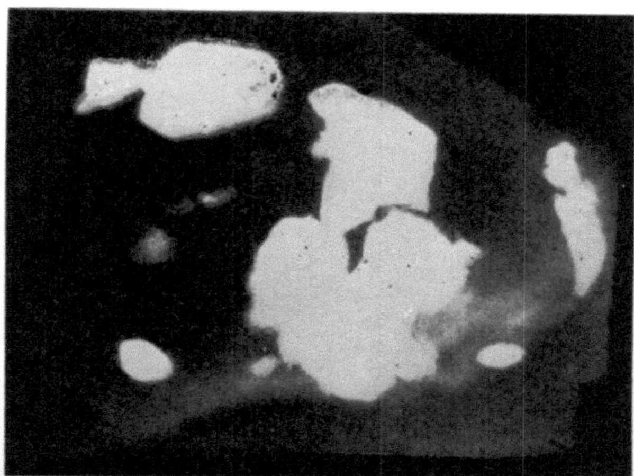

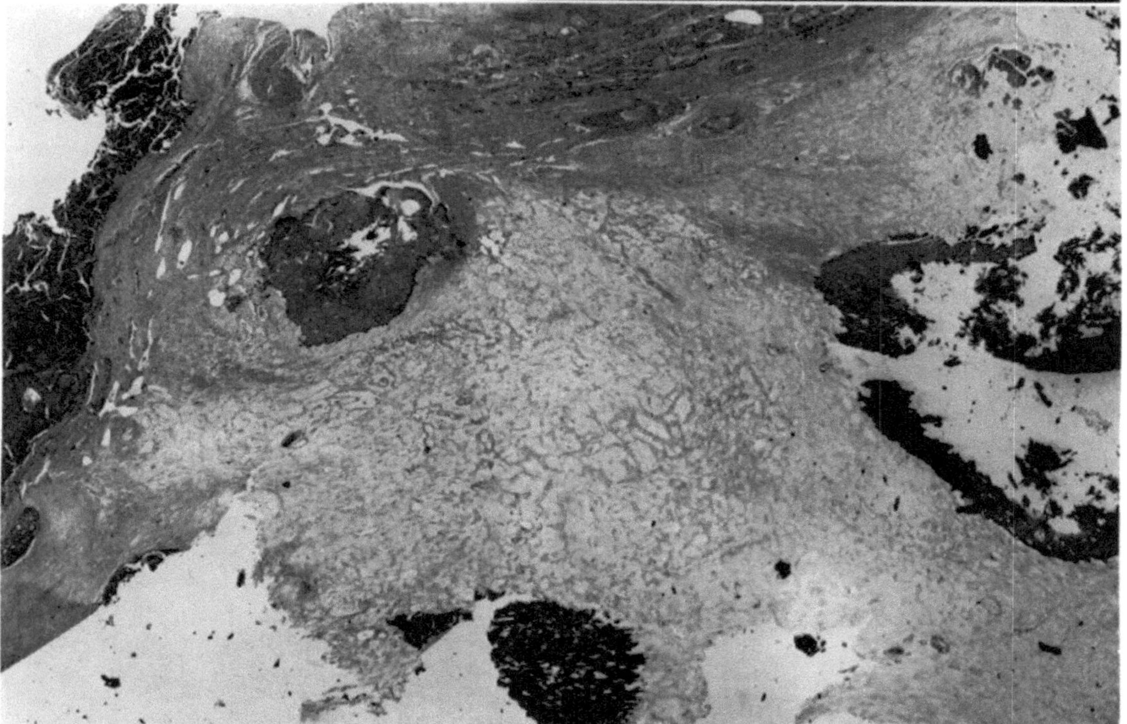

Case 14   Langhans' "wuchernde Struma", a variant of follicular carcinoma, presenting massive calcification. The thyroid tumor consisted of two parts, one being a noncalcified cellular mass and the other a densely calcified fibrous mass with almost completely degenerated tumor cells. Six months following radical neck surgery, pulmonary metastases appeared on the chest x-ray (# 693749, T. S., 48 year-old female).

Fig. 14-a   Roentgenogram of paraffin block specimen (×2.5).

Fig. 14-b   Photomicrograph of specimen. The tumor parenchyma had undergone degenerative change and has been replaced by fibrosis, where extremely dense calcification has occurred. In the extreme left portion, solid proliferation of tumor cells typical of "wuchernde Struma" is seen. (H & E, ×7).

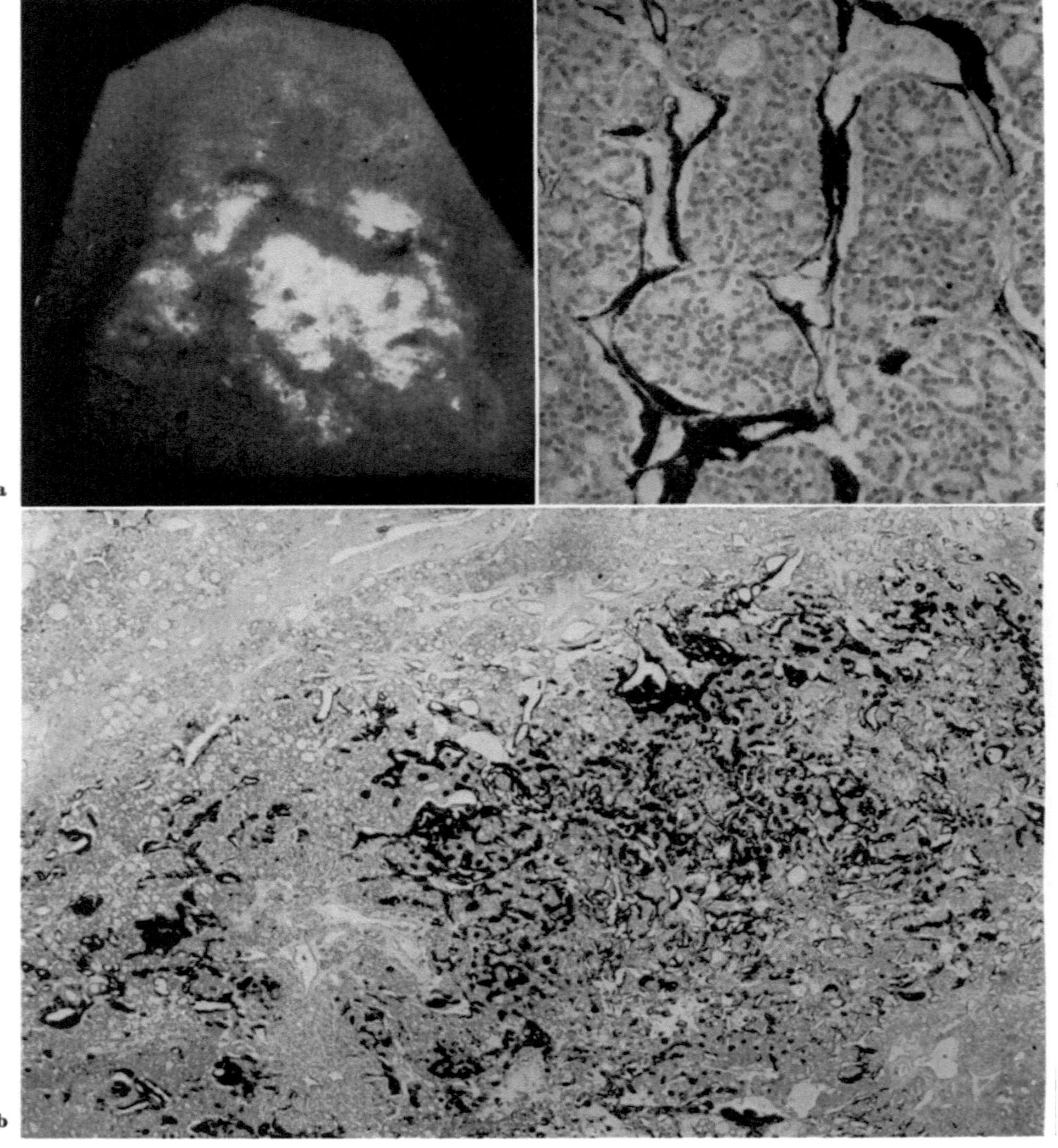

Case 15   Microfollicular adenoma showing a fleece-like pattern of calcification (# 684269, F. K., 46 year-old female)

Fig. 15-a   Roentgenogram of paraffin block specimen, showing a fleece-like pattern of calcification. The shadow is radiologically of low density ($\times$2.5).

Fig. 15-b   Low power photomicrograph of specimen, showing calcium deposits along the sinusoidal vascular structures of the adenoma (Kóssa, $\times$15).

Fig. 15-c   High power view of histologic section (Kóssa, $\times$70).

DIAGNOSTIC SIGNIFICANCE OF THYROID CALCIFICATION

The results of our study on the surgical specimens have led us to the same conclusion as that stated by previous investigators (KLINCK and WINSHIP, 1959; BATSAKIS et al., 1960; HISADA et al., 1962; ONISHI, 1966; HOSHI et al., 1967; MARGOLIN et al., 1967). Namely, only the presence of psammoma bodies is of diagnostic value and they are almost pathognomonic of the thyroid carcinoma.

Psammoma bodies were found histologically in approximately half of the thyroid carcinomas in our series as well as in other investigators' series. The important fact is that the bodies were present in a very few cases of benign thyroid disorders, the incidence being one out of 2,153 noncancerous thyroids in KLINCK's series, 10 out of 612 in BATSAKIS' study, 1.9% of adenomatous goiters and 2.0% of adenomas in HOSHI's study, and only 2 of 98 benign nodules in our series.

It should be kept in mind that the incidences of psammoma bodies cited above are all derived from histological studies. The soft tissue roentgenography of paraffin block specimens gave us a similar incidence of psammomatous calcification. But, as will be stated in the following chapter, psammoma bodies present in about half of the cancer cases and in almost all the cases of benign nodule are small in amount, scattered and non-conglomerated, so that even with the optimal technique now available they are unable to be demonstrated on roentgenograms of the neck. Therefore, psammoma bodies in benign nodules are, as a rule, not demonstrable by roentgenograms. If the psammomatous calcifications are observed on the neck roentgenograms, the finding can be evaluated as a difinitive sign indicative of the presence of thyroid cancer.

Coarse calcifications were, on the other hand, found to have a similar incidence in both benign and malignant lesions in our present series. Furthermore no apparent correlation existed between the configurations of coarse calcific deposits and the histologic diagnoses.

AGE AND SEX DISTRIBUTION OF PATIENTS WITH PAPILLARY CARCINOMA CONTAINING PSAMMOMATOUS CALCIFICATION

It appears to have some diagnostic significance to analyse the age and sex distributions of patients with thyroid carcinoma from the standpoint of the presence or absence of psammomatous calcification. Of 59 cancer patients who were positive for psammomatous calcification in our series, 48 patients or 81% were those with papillary carcinoma. Since the numbers of patients with carcinomas other than papillary carcinoma were not large enough for a biological analysis, only those with papillary carcinoma are considered here.

The papillary carcinoma is the most common type of the thyroid cancer and in our series there were 81 cases (79 papillary carcinomas and 2 papillary combined with anaplastic carcinomas) in a total 100 consecutive cancer patients. Of these 81 papillary carcinomas, 49 or 61% had psammomatous calcification. Their age and sex distributions are shown in Fig. 16.

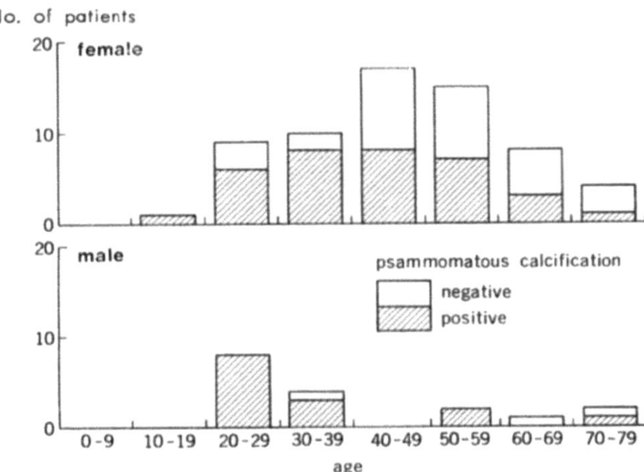

Fig. 16 Sex and age distribution of pateints with papillary carcinoma of the thyroid who are positive or negative for psammomatous calcification.

There were 17 male patients and psammomatous calcification was positive in all but three, who were 30, 64 and 71 years old.   In general, the incidence of psammomatous calcification in female patients was much less, the tendency being more marked in the old patients.   More than half of the female patients who were older than 40 did not contain psammoma bodies.

Chapter III

In Vitro Phantom Experiment

A Basic Study on the Application of Soft Tissue Roentgenography for the Roentgenographic Demonstration of Intrathyroidal Calcification

INTRODUCTION

As stated in the preceding chapter, the diagnostic value of psammoma bodies in thyroid cancer has been confirmed by the histologic and roentgenographic studies on the resected specimens. Then the next important problem to be solved is how to demonstrate psammoma bodies on the roentgenogram of the neck preoperatively.

Several investigators (SEGAL et al., 1960; GASQUET et al., 1963; MARGOLIN and STEINBACH, 1968; and HIGUCHI et al., 1969) have already attempted the clinical use of soft tissue roentgenography in roentgenographic visualization of the faint, tiny calcified bodies. They all agreed that it was a useful diagnostic tool because there were no false positive results, but even with this special technique, psammoma bodies were of insufficient number and density to be identified in a fairly large percentage of patients. These results implied the necessity of the critical review and refinement of the technique.

The paramount aim of soft tissue roentgenography is to provide maximal detail and contrast on roentgenograms. The principles of the technique include the lowest kilovoltage required for penetration, compensation by high milliampere and long exposure time, proper collimation with a cylinder cone, no filtration, short object-to-film distance, fine grain industrial type of film, elimination of intensifying screens and manual processing.

Soft tissue roentgenography has successfully been applied in mammography and at present it is accepted as a reliable diagnostic tool. The breast is actually the most suitable tissue to fulfill the principles of the technique cited above. In contrast to the female breast which contains considerable amount of adipose tissue readily penetrated by x-ray, the anterior half of the neck where the thyroid gland or its pathologic process is located includes neck muscles and great blood vessels which necessitate higher kilovoltage for x-ray penetration. Hence mammography is carried out with the peak kilovoltage (kVp) of 25 to 30 in EGAN's technique (1964), whereas the roentgenogram of the neck has to be taken with 35 to 40 kVp in the oblique projection and 40 to 45 kVp in the lateral projection.

On the roentgenogram of the neck, neither the nodular mass nor the fibrous process within the thyroid gland are demonstrable as a recognizable density. Only the substances with higher density such as calcific deposits are visualized on the films. To achieve a distinct roentgenographic demonstration of psammoma bodies of low radiological density, further refinement would be necessary. One of the factors considered is proper collimation of x-ray beam with the use of a long cylinder cone, although it limits the observation field. Another factor is a proper projection, which includes the least amount of muscles and blood vessels along the course of the central x-ray beam and thus minimizes the production of scattered radiation.

Other principles of soft tissue roentgenography can be applied in the neck study, such as no filtration, short object-to-film distance, fine grain industrial film and its manual processing. As for the use of intensifying screens, the conventional types of screen should be excluded in order to obtain sufficient details on the roentgenograms. However, as will be stated later, an ultrafine type of screen may be worth consideration for shortening the exposure time, if it is proven not to decrease the sharpness of detail.

With these considerations in mind we performed *in vitro* phantom experiments.

MATERIALS AND METHODS

Three paraffin block specimens of surgically removed cancer tissues were chosen as the test materials, which were known to contain psammoma bodies, coarse amorphous calcification and coarse calcific deposit of net-work configulation, respectively (Fig. 17). The first specimen was chosen as it contained psammoma bodies of the nonconglomerated and scattered pattern, which were the most difficult ones to be demonstrated on the roentgenogram. These three specimens were connected in parallel with paraffin and were placed within a neck phantom.

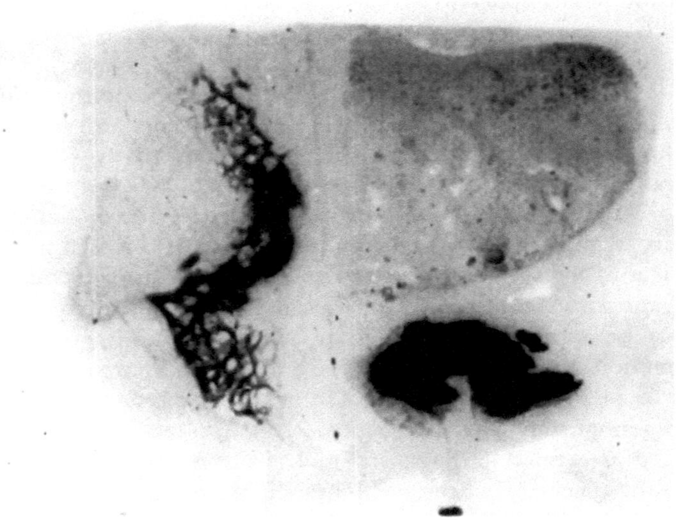

Fig. 17 Roentgenogram of the paraffin block specimens that were used as test materials in a water phantom experiment. All the three specimens were thyroid cancers and contained psammoma bodies (right upper), coarse amorphous calcification (right bottom) and coarse deposit of net-work configulation (left). ($\times$2)

The phantom was made up of two plastic columns and a bottom plate (Fig. 18). A thinner column of 2.6 cm in diameter was set up as a substitute for the trachea within a wider column of 11 cm in diameter and the cavity between the two columns and the bottom was filled with water.

Considerable experimentation was carried out in the following three procedures, each with a variety of technical factors.

1. Lateral projection with a use of standard roentgenographic technique.
2. Lateral projection with soft tissue technique (Fig. 19A).
3. Tangential projection with soft tissue technique using a long cylinder extension cone, 4.5 cm in diameter and 35 cm in length (Fig. 18B). This projection is hereafter referred to as the "spot-tangential" projection.

Rotating anode x-ray tube for mammography type DRX-20A (Toshiba)* was used. The range of technical factors applied in each projection and those found optimal are shown in Table 5.

The main differences between the first and the second procedures are: 65 kVp, 200 mA, and medical film with FS type of intensifying screen in the former, as compared to 40–45 kVp, 150 mA, fine

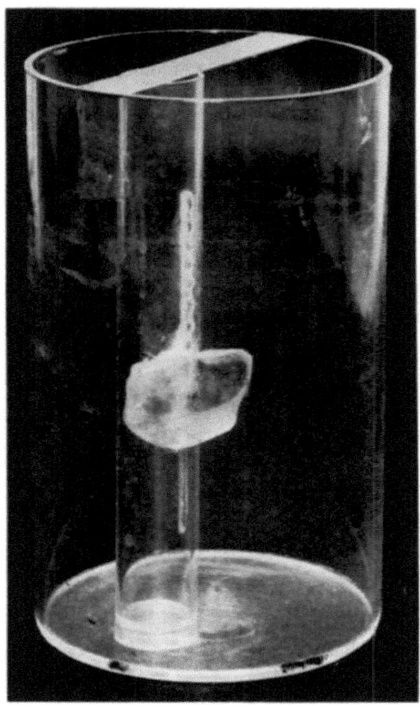

Fig. 18 Neck phantom.

Table 5 Range of Technical Factors Used for Water Phantom Experiment.

Projection	Technical Factors
1. Lateral projection, ordinary roentgenogram	65 kVp, 200 mA, 0.05 sec., Focal-film distance 150 cm, Intensifying screen Type FS, Multi-leaf shutter, Medical film, No Bucky.
2. Lateral projection, soft tissue roentgenogram	30–45 (optimal 40–45) kVp, 150 mA, 1.5–2.5 (optimal 1.5–2.0) sec., Focal-object distance 42 cm, No screens, Diversing cone[a], Fine grain industrial film, No Bucky.
3. Spot-tangential projection, soft tissue roentgenogram	30–45 (optimal 35–40) kVp, 150 mA, 1.5–2.5 (optimal 1.5–2.0) sec., Focal-object distance 42 cm, No screens, Cylinder cone[b], Fine grain industrial film, No Bucky.

[a] A diversing cone; proximal diameter 5 cm, distal diameter 10 cm and length 15 cm.

[b] A cylinder cone: diameter 4.5 cm and length 35 cm.

grain industrial film without intensifying screen in the latter. The main differences between the second and the third procedures lie in: 40–45 kVp, lateral projection with a shorter and wider extension cone (diversing cone) in the former, whereas slightly lower kVp of 35 to 40, tangential projection with a longer and narrower extension cone in the latter.

---

* Tokyo Shibaura Electric Co. (Tokyo, Japan)

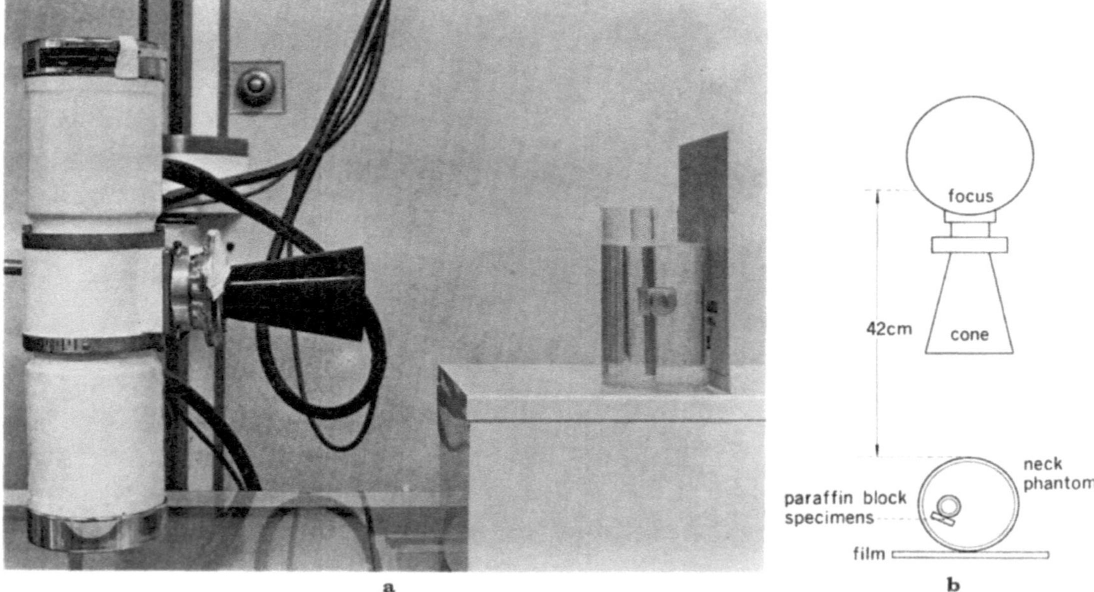

Fig. 19 A   Positioning for the lateral view with the use of soft tissue roentgenography, seen from the side (a) and from above (b).

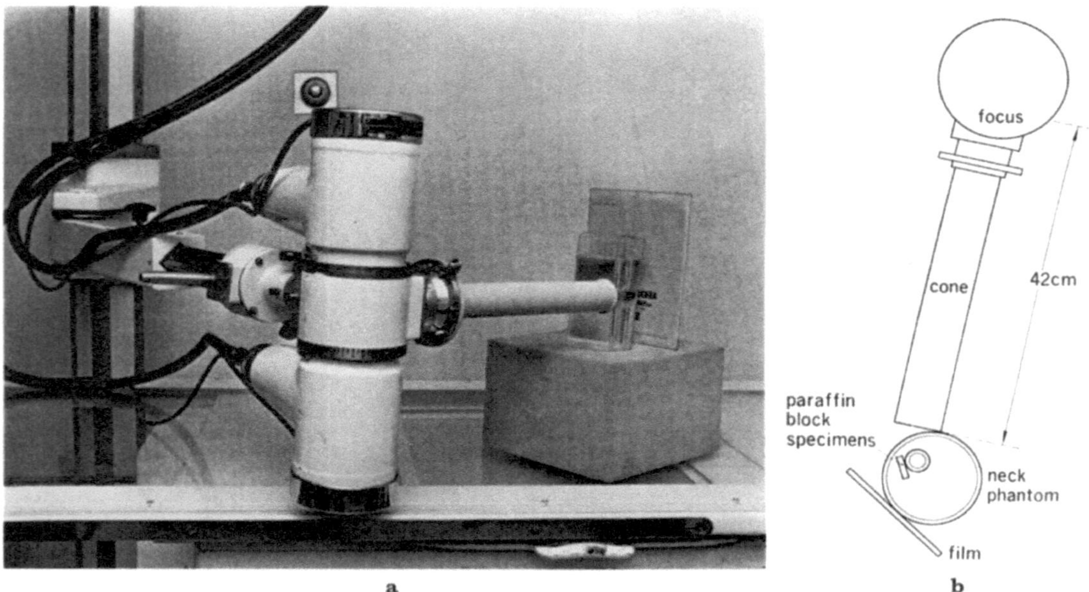

Fig. 19 B   Positioning for the spot-tangential view with the use of soft tissue roentgenography, seen from the side (a) and from above (b).

RESULTS AND COMMENTS

The three different patterns of calcifications demonstrated on the roentgenograms were critically reviewed as to quality with respect to the contrast, sharpness of detail and image resolution.

a. Coarse Calcific Deposits

The shadows of coarse calcific deposits were recognizable by all the three roentgenographic procedures (Fig. 20, 21 and 22). However, as for detail, roentgenograms obtained by the second and third procedure which used the technique of soft tissue roentgenography were far superior to the one obtained by standard roentgenography. Comparing the two procedures of soft tissue roentgenography, shadows of coarse calcific deposits on the lateral view taken by the second procedure were roentgenologically slightly inferior, but clinically satisfactory for diagnostic use. Taking into consideration the great advantage of obtaining a wider area on the roentgenogram of the second procedure, we may conclude that, for a demonstration of coarse calcific deposits, the lateral projection covering the whole anterior part of the neck with the technique of soft tissue roentgenography is the method of choice.

b. Psammoma Bodies

The main purpose of this phantom study was the development of a technique which would allow the roentgenographic demonstration of psmamoma bodies.

In general, the lateral projection with the use of standard roentgenography is completely unsatisfactory in this respect. When psammoma bodies are present in non-conglomerated form and are scattered as in the test specimen, they are absolutely undetectable on the roentgenograms (Fig. 20).

Psammoma bodies were demonstrated on both the lateral and the spot-tangential views of soft tissue roentgenography (Fig. 21 and 22). When these two views were compared, the latter produced a better image with respect to contrast, detail and image resolution. Thus our approach with strict adherence to the principles of soft tissue roentgenography in an attempt to demonstrate psammoma bodies was verified in this phantom experiment.

In the clinical application of this soft tissue roentgenography, the neck roentgenograms obtained were of slightly inferior quality, and therefore the results of the water phantom experiment were retrospectively reviewed. We recognized the fact that the tissue specimen produced better contrast because it was sliced and imbedded in paraffin which was more radiolucent than water. In addition, the water phantom was absolutely motionless during the exposure, whereas some motion was inevitable in neck roentgenography.

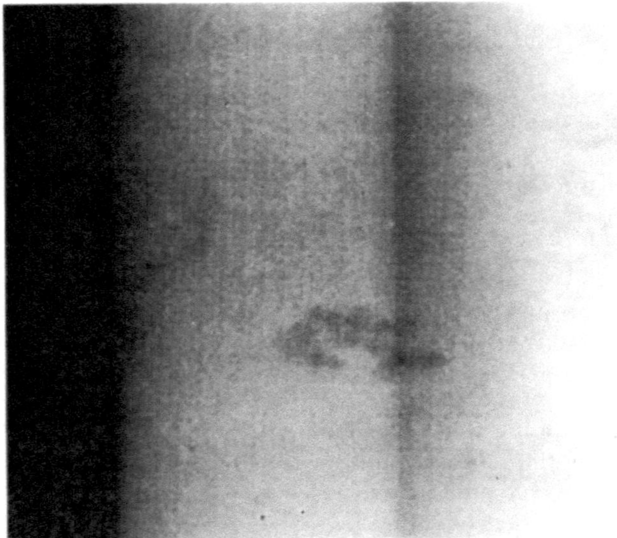

Fig. 20 Lateral view of the water phantom taken by the technique of oridinary roentgenography. Technical factors were: 65 kVp, 200 mA, 0.05 sec., focal-film distance 150 cm, intensifying screen Type FS, multi-leaf shutter, medical film and no Bucky. Coarse calcific deposits were demonstrated on the film, but psammoma bodies could not be identified. (×2)

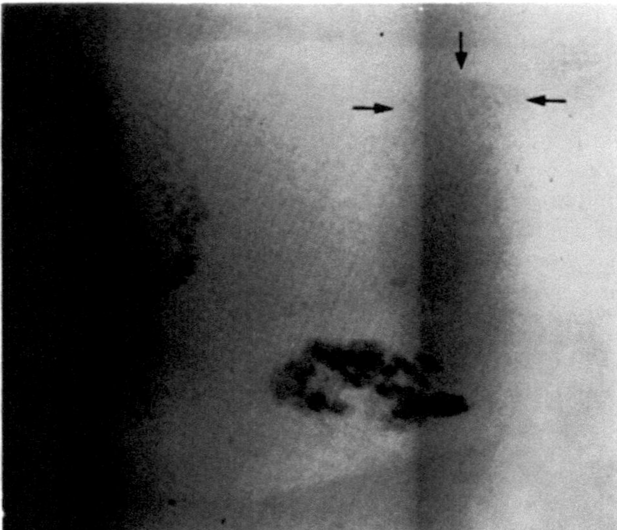

Fig. 21 Lateral view of the phantom taken with the soft tissue technique. Technical factors were: 40 kVp, 150 mA, 1.5 sec., focal-object distance 42 cm, no screen, diversing cone, industrial film and no Bucky. All the three types of calcification were shown on the film. (×2)

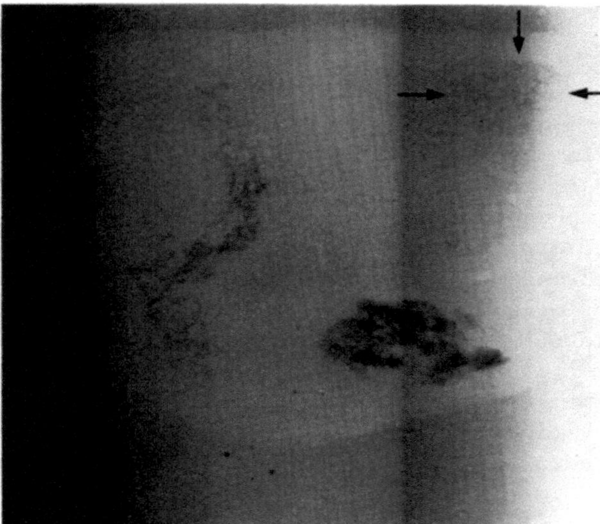

Fig. 22 Spot-tangential view of the phantom taken by the technique of soft-tissue roentgenography. Technical factors were: 35 kVp, 150 mA, 1.5 sec., focal-object distance 42 cm, no screen, cylinder cone, industrial film and no Bucky. Psammoma bodies are very well shown on the film. (×2)

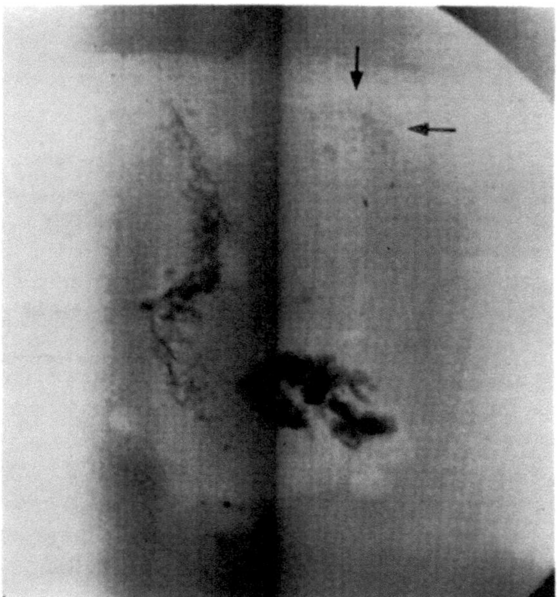

Fig. 23 Spot-tangential view of the phantom obtained by soft tissue roentgeno-graphy with the same technical factors as applied for the roentgenogram shown in Fig. 23, except for an exposure time 0.8 sec. and the application of ultrafine intensifying screen Type BS. (×2)

RADIATION DOSAGE TO THE SKIN

When compared to conventional roentgenography, the technique of soft tissue roentgenography has the disadvantage of increased radiation dosage to the exposed skin.

Measurements of the skin dose were made in each procedure using Siemens' universal dosimeter, with the technical factors necessary to obtain the film density of 1.0. The dosage with the lateral projection using standard roentgenography was 0.3 R, whereas soft tissue roentgenography gave comparatively large values at the exposed skin with lateral projection and tangential projection of approximately 6 R and 9 R, respectively. These values are comparable to those of mammography. EGAN (1964) reported 2.4 to 6.5 rads with craniocaudad projection of mammography, which was done with lower kilovoltage ranging from 25 to 30 kVp. When one of the authors (M. A.) (1966) investigated skin dose at mammography, it was found to be 6.5 R with the technical factors commonly used for young adults: 30 kVp, focal-skin distance of 40 cm, 150 mA and 2.0 sec., and 4.7 R with the factors for older women: 28 kVp, focal-skin distance of 40 cm, 150 mA and 1.5 sec.

Although the x-ray is focused only at the anterolateral portion of the neck and the radiation hazard to the gonads appears to be negligible, it is needless to say that the least amount of exposure is desirable. Our endeavors have been in that direction. Recently we considered the application of intensifying screens. However, thus far an intensifying screen has not generally been used in the soft tissue roentgenography because of the decreased image resolution. But it was proved that a 50 percent decrease in the radiation dosage was attained with the use of an ultrafine intensifying screen (Type BS Kyokko, Dainihon Toryo Co., Ltd.*), without compromising the quality of roentgenograms. The details will be described in the following paragraph.

TECHNICAL REFINEMENT

As is well known to radiologists who have experience in soft tissue roentgenography, a long exposure time and the resulting motion blur are inevitable even in the cooperative patient. When an ultrafine intensifying screen is applied to the film, reduction of exposure time by 50 percent is possible. In addition, it has the advantage of decreasing radiation dosage to the patient as described above. This method provides better image contrast with negligible compromise of image resolution (Fig. 24).

When using intensifying screens, it is important to obtain perfect film-screen contact and also to avoid screens having any minute defects, which may produce artifacts simulating psammomatous calcifications.

As to the target, GROS (1967) and GERSHON-COHEN et al. (1970) have adopted a molybdenum target in mammography, whose K radiation wave-edge length is 0.7 Å, in contrast to 0.2 Å for tangsten. Recently we began to employ a similar molybdenum target in the neck roentgenography. This target has provided roentgenograms of superior image resolution.

---

* Dainihon Toryo Co. Ltd., Odawara, Japan

Chapter IV

Roentgenographic Technique

In patients with nodular disorders of the thyroid three projections of the neck are routinely taken.

1. A standard roentgenogram in the anteroposterior projection.
2. Soft tissue roentgenogram in the lateral projection.
3. Soft tissue roentgenogram in the spot-tangential projection.

The latter two views are important in the examination for intrathyroidal calcification. The technical factors applied to the average patient in each projection are listed in Table 6.

Table 6 Technical Factors Used in Roentgenograms of the Neck.

Projection	Technical Factors
1. Antero-posterior projection, standard roentgenogram	78 kVp, 200 mA, 0.16 sec., Focal-film distance 150 cm, Intensifying screen Type FS, Multi-leaf shutter, Medical film, Bucky 5 : 1.
2. Lateral projection, soft tissue roentgenogram	40–45 kVp, 150 mA, 1.5–2.0 sec., Focal-skin distance 42 cm, No intensifying screen, Diverging cone, Industrial film, No Bucky.
3. Spot-tangential projection, soft tissue roentgenogram	35–40 kVp, 150 mA, 1.5–2.0 sec., Focal-skin distance 42 cm, No intensifying screen, Cylinder cone*, Industrial film, No Bucky.

* See the footnotes in Table 5.

A medical film is used for standard roentgenography and a fine grain industrial film is used for soft tissue roentgenography. For the latter, we have used Sakura X-Ray Film, Type MR, or Fuji Mammography Envelope Pack, but Kodak Industrial X-ray Film, Type M or recently developed Kodak X-ray Film Type RP/M are also available.

A film of 20×25.5 cm in size is needed for the lateral view. The spot-tangential view can be taken on a 12×16.5 cm film. When more than two spot-tangential projections are taken in the same patient, as for an extremely large nodule or multiple nodules in the both lobes of the thyroid, a 20×25.5 cm sheet of film can be used to include all the views, or smaller sheets of film can be used for each projection.

It must be recognized that the water phantom remains absolutely still during the long exposure time, whereas some motion blur is inevitable in clinical roentgenography. Extreme care should be exercised to minimize this motion. To accomplish this, the patient must be relaxed and be placed in a comfortable position. Breathing is held during the exposure. Even in cooperative patients, motion from vascular pulsation can not be avoided.

As recommended by STANTON and LIGHTFOOT (1966), some increase in visual contrast is achieved by simply exposing roentgenograms at a slightly higher kilovoltage(2 to 3 kV) than usual to increase film density.   The darker film is then viewed with good masking on a bright adjustable-intensity view box.   This is especially true with the soft tissue roentgenographs.

ANTERO-POSTERIOR PROJECTION STANDARD ROENTGENOGRAM

This is the same method as conventionally used for roentgenologic examination of the larynx, trachea and cervical spine.   Although the posteroanterior projection is theoretically indicated for the roentgenologic examination of the thyroid which places the gland closer to the film, the anteroposterior projection is usually obtained.   This is because the positioning for the latter exposure is easier and only the clear delineation of the tracheal air column is desired in this view.

For the anteroposterior projection, the patient sits on a chair in front of the film holder, with her occiput and back in contact with the film cassette (Fig. 24).   The chin is held slightly upward and the anterior part of the neck is extended.

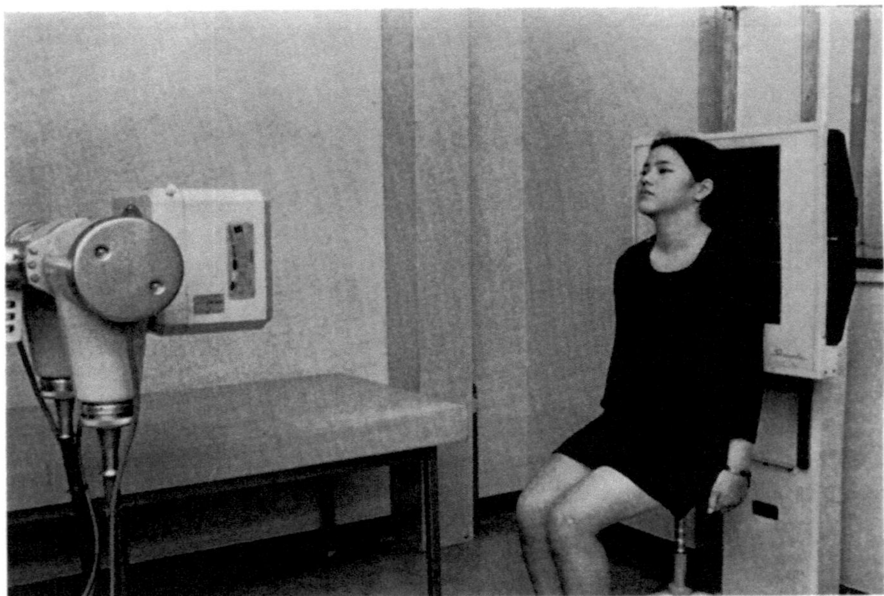

Fig. 24   Positioning for the antero-posterior projection with the standard roentgenographic technique. The patient is seated, the occiput and back in contact with the film cassette and the chin held slightly upward.   Technical factors for the average pateints are: 78 kVp, 200 mA, 0.16 sec., focal-film distance of 150 cm, intensifying screen Type FS, multi-leaf shutter, medical film and Bucky 5: 1.

This projection permits study of displacement and compression of the trachea from either side caused by the enlarged thyroid.   Indentation or invasion, if present, can be observed.   In general, the anteroposterior view is not suitable for demonstration of intrathyroidal calcification, because even if calcific shadows are actually present, they are obscured by the superimposed cervical spine.   Only coarse calcific deposits in enormous thyroid nodules can be shown extending beyond the spinal shadow.

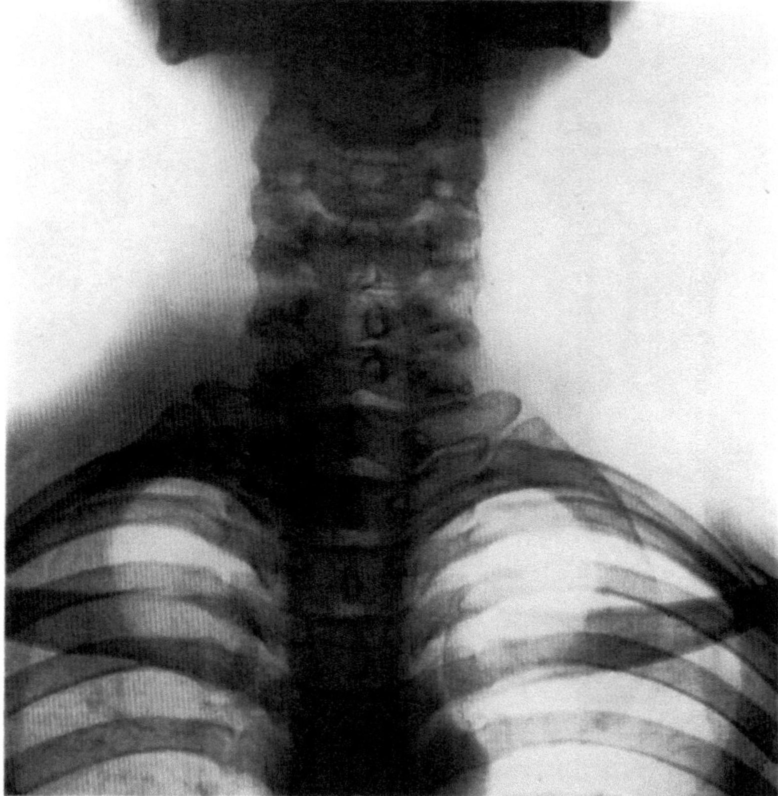

Fig. 25   An example of a standard roentgenogram of the neck:
antero-posterior projection.

LATERAL PROJECTION SOFT TISSUE ROENTGENOGRAM

The patient is placed in a lateral or a slightly prone position on the roentgenographic table with the side of interest down.   The lower shoulder is pulled back with the arm being placed behind the back.   A pillow is inserted under the head and neck and pre-packed film is placed between the neck and the pillow (Fig. 26 a and b).   Thus the lateral aspect of the neck and a portion of the anterolateral aspect of the upper thorax are brought in contact with the film. The tube with its diverging cone is then angulated 90 degrees toward a saggital plane of the neck.   Although this positioning can provide close contact of the film to the neck skin, the film is flexed fairly sharply between the pillow and the clavicle and therefore the thyroid lesion, if present in the lower neck, may be shown in an extremely deformed configulation.

In an another position illustrated in Fig. 27, a prepacked film is placed flat on the roentgenographic table and the patient's head is supported on a pillow.   There is some separation between the neck and the film, but this positioning has the advantage of visualization of the entire anterior portion of the neck and allows evaluation of a lesion in relation to the surrounding tissue without distortion.

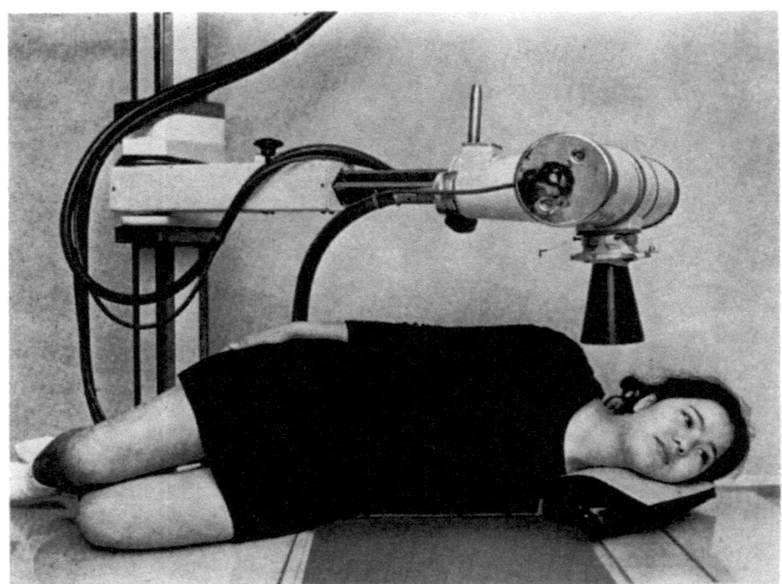

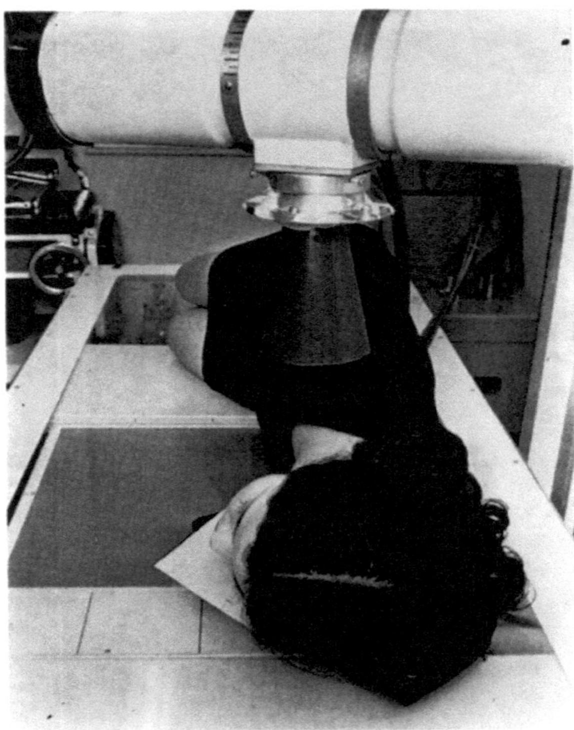

Fig. 26   Positioning for the lateral view with the use of soft tissue roentgenography, seen from the side
(a) and from above (b).   The patient is placed in a lateral or a slightly prone position on the table
with the desired side down, the lower shoulder pulled back and the lower arm placed behind the back.
A pillow is inserted under the head and neck.   A prepacked film is inserted between the neck and the
pillow.   Technical factors are: 40–45 kVp, 150 mA, 1.5–2.0 sec., focal-skin distance 42 cm, no screen,
diversing cone, industrial film and no Bucky.

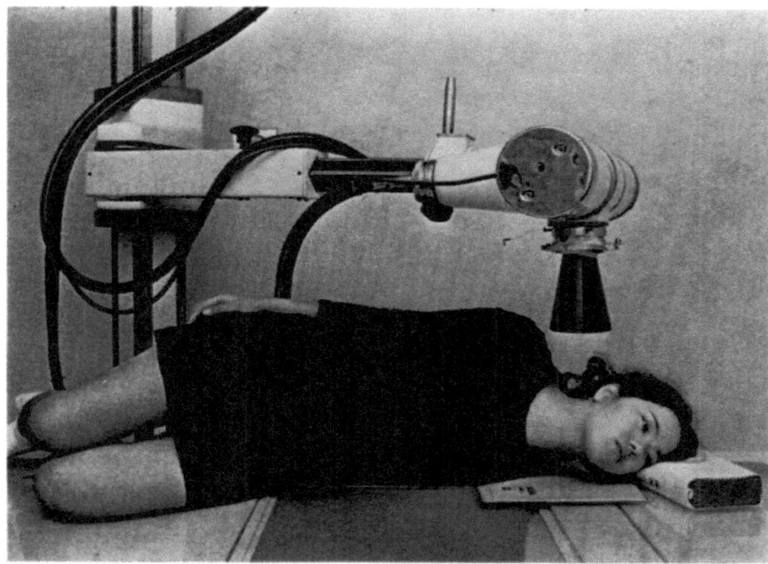

Fig. 27 Another position for the lateral view. A prepacked film is placed flat on the table and the head of the patient is supported by a pillow. Technical factors are the same as those applied in the positioning shown in Fig. 25. This positioning is suitable for demonstrating the entire area of the anterior neck without distortion.

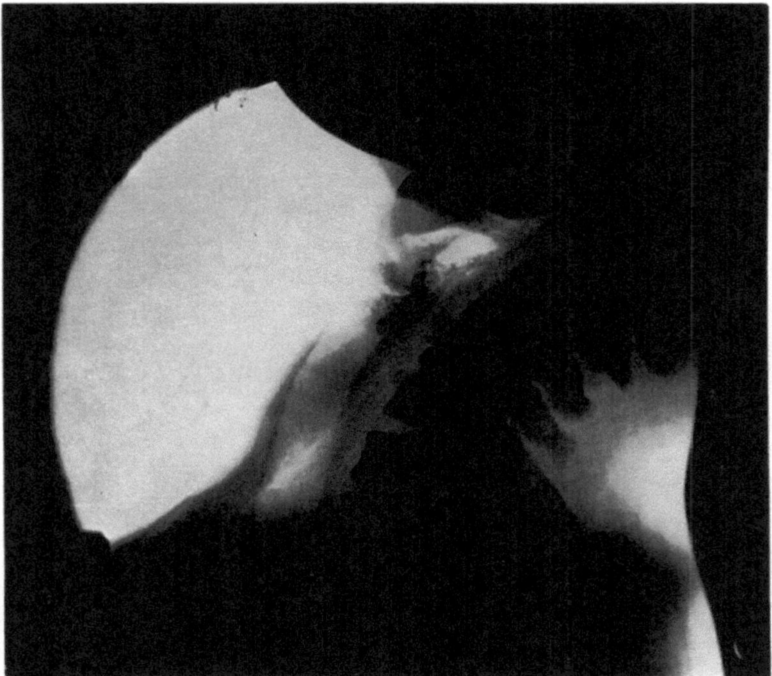

Fig. 28 An example of a soft tissue roentgenogram of the neck: lateral projection. This roentgenogram was taken by the position thown in Fig. 26.

SPOT-TANGENTIAL PROJECTION SOFT TISSUE ROENTGENOGRAM

This is the clinical application of the method that has proved to be the most satisfactory procedure to demonstrate psammoma bodies in *in vitro* phantom experiments.

The aim of this projection is preservation of maximum detail on roentgenograms. However, since only a narrow area is exposed on the roentgenogram, the calcified process may be missed. Exact focusing on the thyroid nodule is extremely important. It is strongly recommended that the physician marks the skin indicating the center of the nodule, so that the technician can achieve the proper projection.

Spot-tangential projection is obtained in one of the following positionings, depending on the location, size and shape of the thyroid nodule.

(a) The patient lies on the roentgenographic table in the semiprone position with the desired side up and with her head and neck on an obliquely placed pillow. A prepacked film is inserted between the neck and the pillow. The anterior end of the pillow is held by the patient in order to prevent motion. Then the tube with its long extension cone is angulated so that the central x-ray beam projects tangentially through the thyroid nodule from the posterolateral side of the neck. The end of the extension cone is brought into close contact with the skin overlying the thyroid nodule (Fig. 30 a and b.).

(b) The patient is placed on the table in the lateral position with the desired side down. The position of head and neck, pillow and prepacked film is the same as stated above. The x-ray beam is projected in an anterior to posterolateral direction (Fig. 31), thus obtaining a tangential projection of the nodule.

(c) When the nodule is located in the isthmus, the patient is placed in the semi-prone position on the table with the anterolateral aspect of the neck brought in contact with the film. The tube is angulated about 30 degrees and a tangential projection is obtained (Fig. 32 a and b).

All the above statements are those applied to the average patient. Technical factors, such as positioning of the patient and the film, tube angulation and exposure factors may have to be adjusted in the individual case.

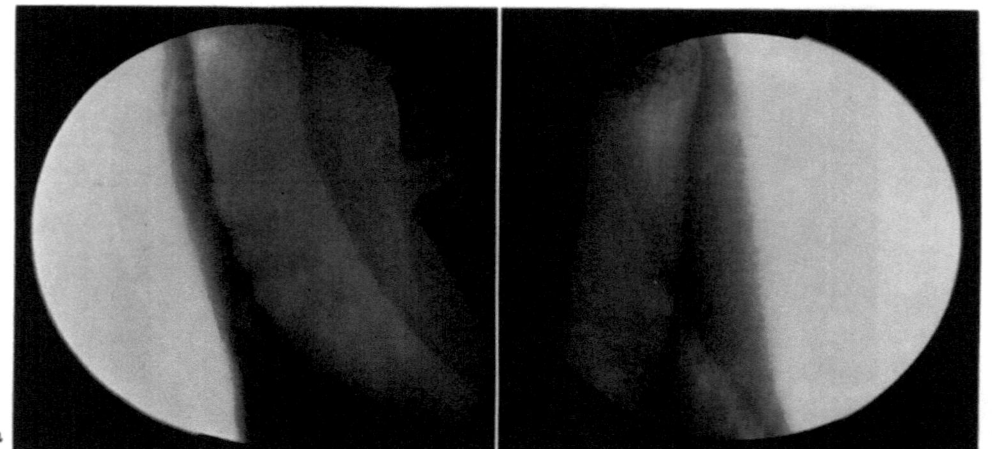

Fig. 29 a, b   Examples of soft tissue roentgenogram of the thyroid region: spot-tangential projection.

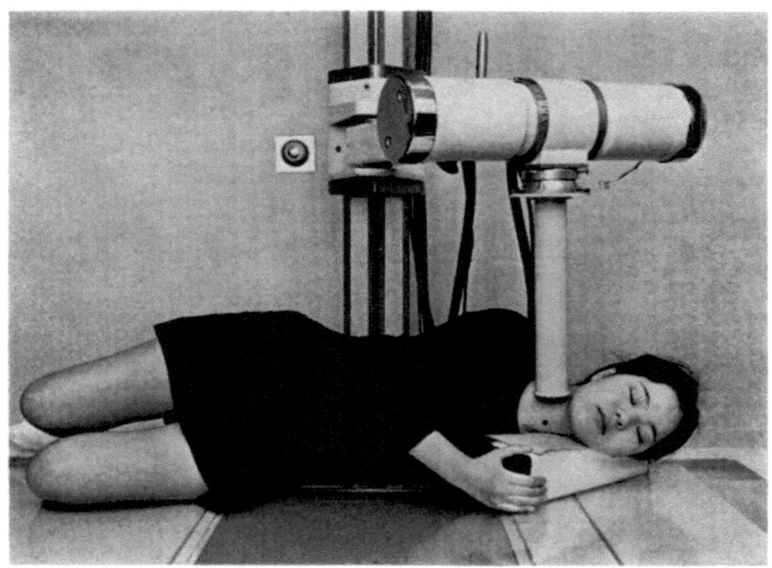

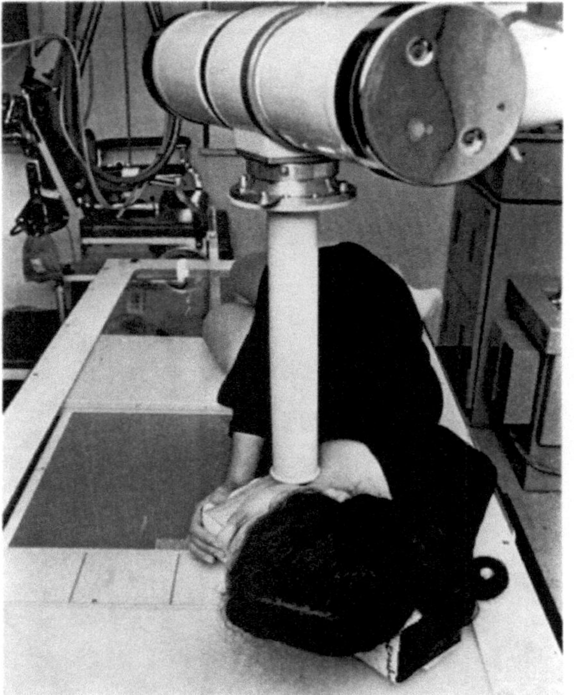

Fig. 30 Positioning for the spot-tangential view of the neck seen from the side (a) and from above (b). The nodule is in the right lobe of the thyroid. The patient is placed on the table in a semi-prone position with the desired side up, the lower shoulder pulled back, the head and neck resting on an obliquely placed pillow, and a prepacked film inserted between the neck and the pillow. The tube with its extension cone is angulated so that the central x-ray beam projects tangentially through the thyroid nodule from the postero-lateral side of the neck. Technical factors are: 35–40 kVp, 150 mA, 1.5–2.0 sec., focal-skin distance 42 cm, industrial film, no screen and no Bucky.

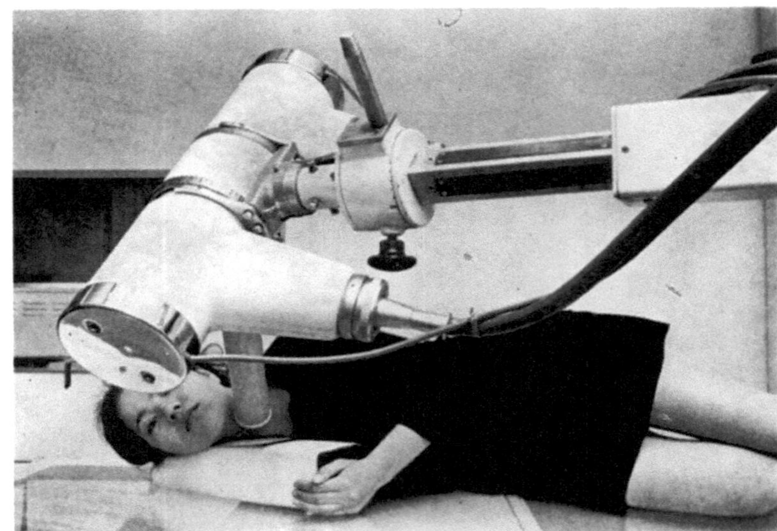

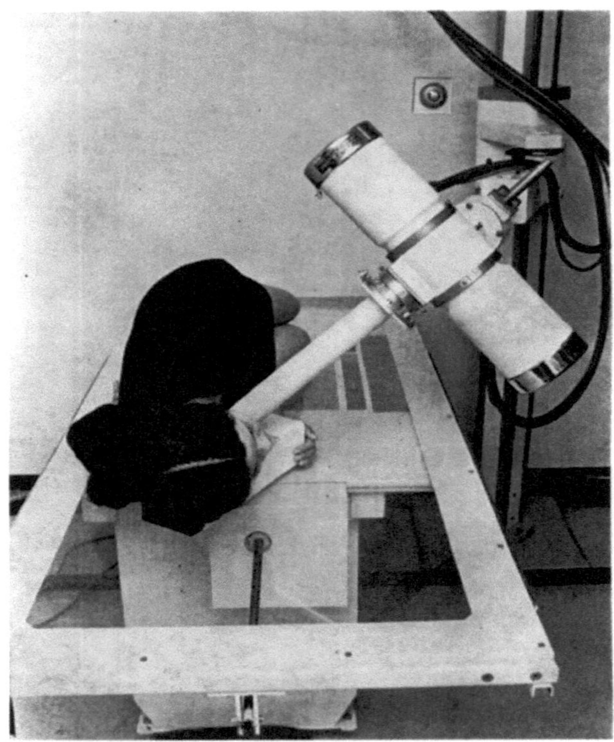

Fig. 31 Another method of positioning for the spot-tangential view of the thyroid nodule locating in the right lobe of the thyroid.   The patient is placed on the table in the lateral position with the desired side down.   The x-ray beam is projected from anterior in a posterolateral direction, so that a tangential projection of the nodule is obtained.   Technical factors are the same as shown in Fig. 30.

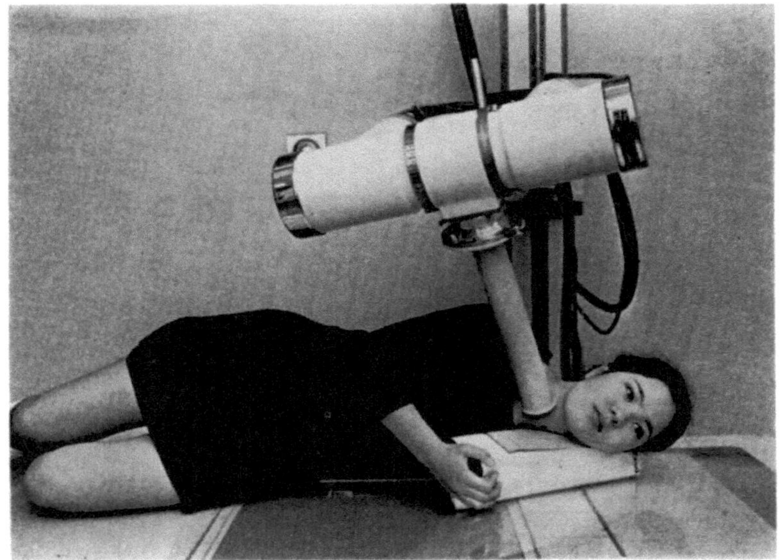

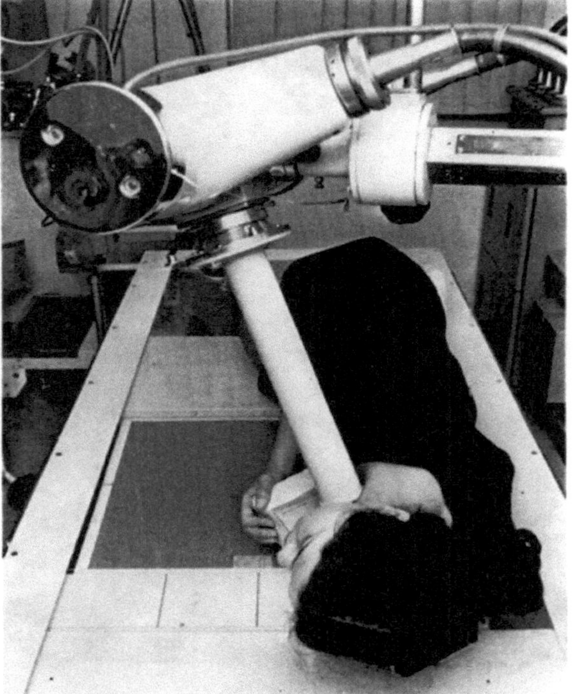

Fig. 32 Positioning for the spot-tangential projection when the nodule is located in the isthmus. The patient is placed in the semi-prone position on the table. The tube with its extension cone is angulated about 30 degrees. Technical factors are the same as shown in Fig. 30.

Chapter V

Roentgenographic Anatomy of the Neck

In the interpretation of neck roentgenograms, complete understanding of the roentgenographic anatomy is important. A variety of anatomical structures with different radiologic densities are shown on a lateral view of the neck. Because of their calcific density, the hyoid bone and ossified cartilages of the larynx are readily identified and, on the other hand, the pharyngo-laryngo-tracheal lumen is visualized as an air-filled clear space.

LOCATION OF THE THYROID GLAND AND ITS PATHOLOGICAL PROCESSES

The thyroid gland partially encases the cervical trachea and larynx. In the normal subjects, the upper pole of the lateral lobe of the thyroid is located at about the mid level of the thyroid cartilage, and the lower pole is 4 to 5 cm below the upper pole. It is well to remember that in females the thyroid cartilage is usually situated in the upper half of the anterior neck and in males, especially in the old persons, it is located at the middle of the neck or even lower. Consequently the thyroid cancers frequently appear comparatively high in the neck in the female patients and rather low in the males.

On the lateral view of the neck, the isthmus of the thyroid is located anterior to the trachea. Occasionally thyroid neoplasm originates in the pyramidal lobe or rarely in the remnant of the thyroglossal duct, which is projected on the roentgenogram just anterior to the larynx or in the thyro-hyoid space.

OSSIFICATION OF LARYNGEAL CARTILAGES

For beginners, the ossified laryngeal cartilages are often confused with calcific deposits within the thyroid. They should be clearly differentiated. The understanding of the exact position of cartilaginous framework of the larynx and its configuration when ossified is a necessity for the roentgenologist.

Among the laryngeal cartilages, the thyroid, cricoid and the greater part of the arythenoid cartilages undergo ossification and two other paired cartilages, the corniculate and cuneiform, do not. Ossification starts during adolescence or young adult life. According to Scheier's opinion (1901), ossification occasionally begins even before the age of 18 years. In general, the process is manifested in the thyroid cartilage first, and shortly thereafter it starts in the cricoid, which is followed by the arythenoid.

Although there are many variations in the mode of ossification in these cartilages, Mittermaier (1970) described the general trends, which are somewhat different according to sex. In males (Figs. 33 a, b), ossification in the thyroid cartilage begins on the anterior edge and also in the region of the inferior cornua. From the latter region it proceeds anteriorly along the inferior margin of the thyroid cartilage and unites with a new bony nucleus which has developed there. The ossification along the inferior margin

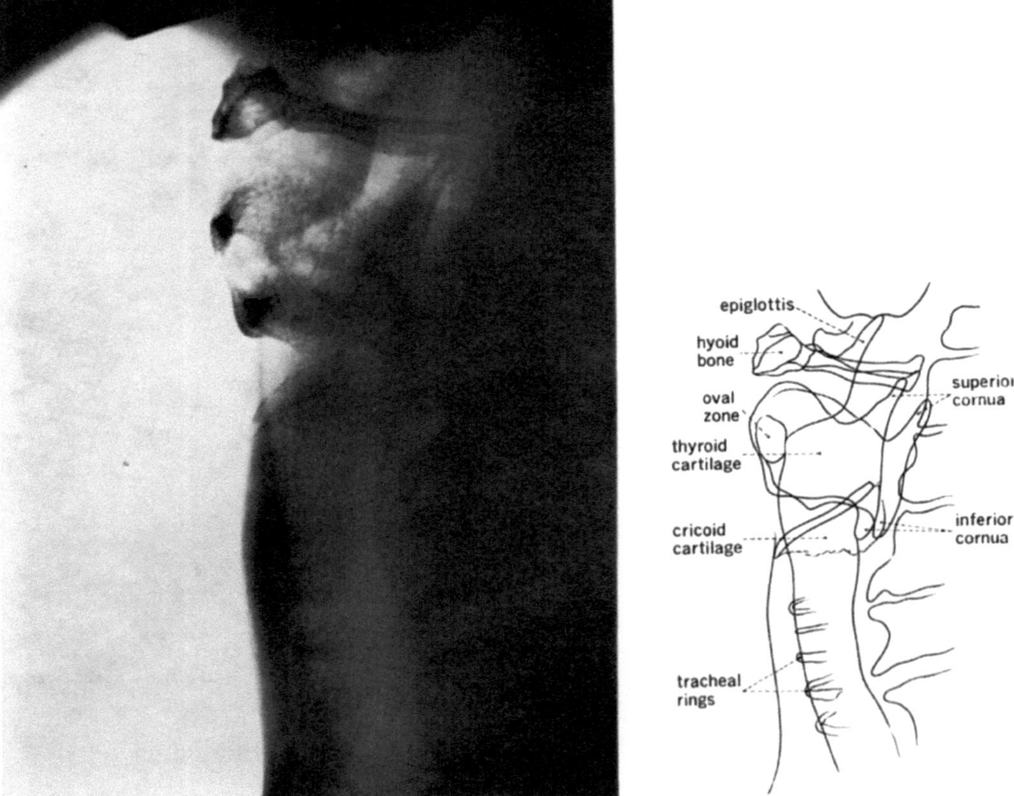

Fig. 33 a Lateral view of the neck to show ossification of laryngeal cartilages. A forty-eight year-old male. Diffusely ossified thyroid and cricoid cartilages are seen. The thyroid cartilage has oval zones which have not ossified. Ossified tracheal rings are also observed.

then progresses all the way to the anterior and superior margins, and finally the upper edges and the superior cornua are ossified, leaving an oval unossified zone on each side. The ossification of the cricoid cartilage starts in its plate. With further ossification the cricoid arches are seen as oblique narrow bony structures on the lateral neck roentgenogram. The superior margin of the cricoid arch is crossed by the inferior margin of the thyroid cartilage.

In females (Figs. 34 a, b), ossification tends to start somewhat later in life and involves smaller areas than in males. The latter fact is well shown in the thyroid cartilage, in which ossification starts in the inferior cornua and progresses anteriorly along the inferior margin, but actually it is rare that the ossification zone reaches the anterior margin of the thyroid plate. The ossification in the cricoid and the arythenoid cartilages proceeds in the similar fashion to that in males.

In both sexes, the inferior cornua of the thyroid cartilage are almost superimposed over the plate of the cricoid cartilage. The arythenoid cartilages are usually shown as denser shadows along the posterior edge of laryngeal cartilagenous framework (Fig. 34).

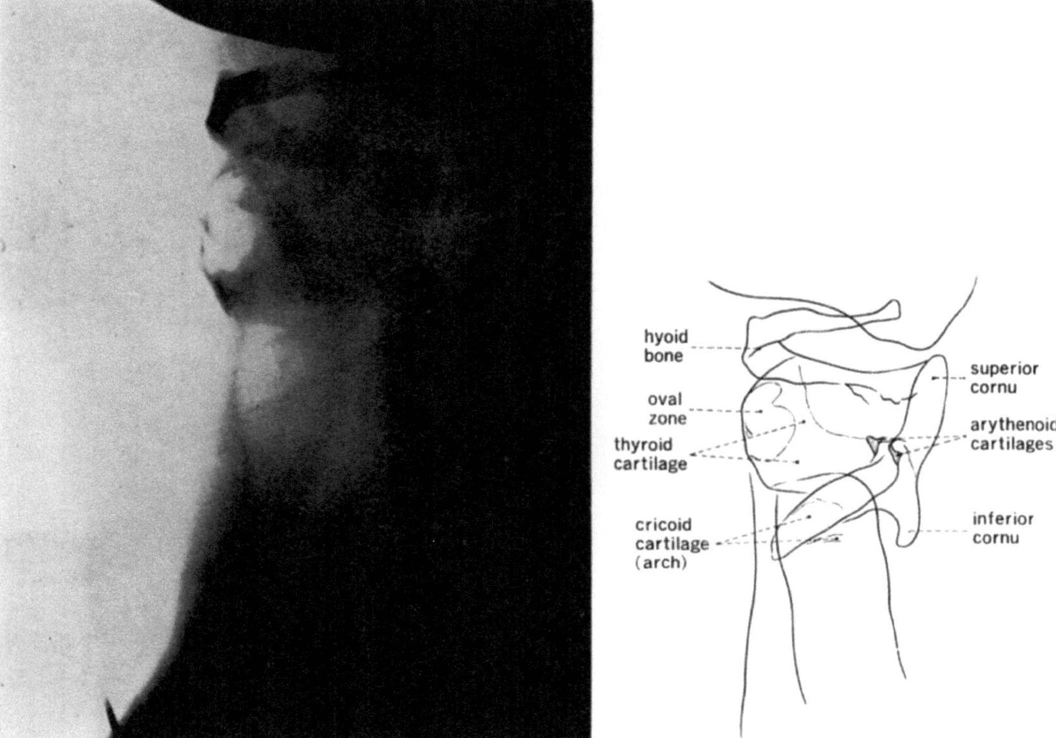

Fig. 33 b Lateral view of the neck taken in a thirty-eight year-old male. In the thyroid cartilarge, ossification has occurred in the superior and inferior cornua, the lower margin and the anterior edge, leaving the superior edge and oval zones unossified. In the cricoid cartilage, the plate and the superior margins of the arch are ossified.

CALCIFIC SHADOWS WHICH NEED DIFFERENTIATION FROM INTRATHYROIDAL CALCIFICATION

As stated above, ossified cartilages of the larynx should not be confused with the calcific deposits within the thyroid gland. When the nodule in the upper part of the thyroid lobe actually has calcific deposits, their shadows are difficult to identify on the roentgenogram, because of their superimposition on the ossified cricoid and thyroid cartilages. In such case, careful study of the outlines of the inferior cornua of the thyroid cartilage, the cricoid plate and arches, and the arythenoid cartilages may lead to the identification of abnormal calcific shadows produced by thyroid disease.

There are other physiological as well as pathological processes that produce calcific shadows on the neck roentgenograms, such as calcified tracheal rings, lymph nodes, blood vessels and ligaments. All these are of a coarse pattern. Calcified tracheal rings appear as transverse band-like shadows on the tracheal air column (Figs. 33a, 34a). Calcified cervical lymph nodes appear mostly in the retrolaryngeal space, which are frequently due to tubercular adenitis, but occasionally due to metastatic lesions from thyroid cancer. Vascular calcifications are seen in the carotid arteries. Along the cervical spine, calcification of the anterior longitudinal ligament or at sites of osteochondrosis may be observed, but these calcific shadows are usually not confused with those occuring within the thyroid.

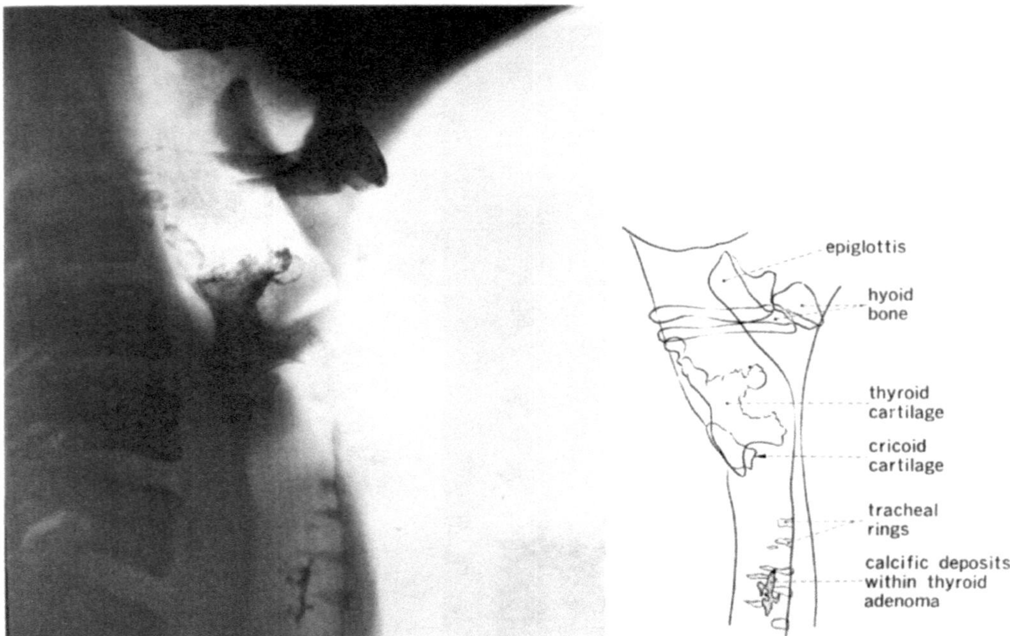

Fig. 34 a   Lateral view of the neck taken in a forty-five year-old female. Ossification of the thyroid cartilage is apparent in the posterior and inferior portions. The cricoid cartilage is also ossified in its plate and the posterior parts of the arch. Ossification has occurred in the tracheal rings. The coarse amorphous shadow superimposed on the tracheal air space is due to a calcified adenoma.

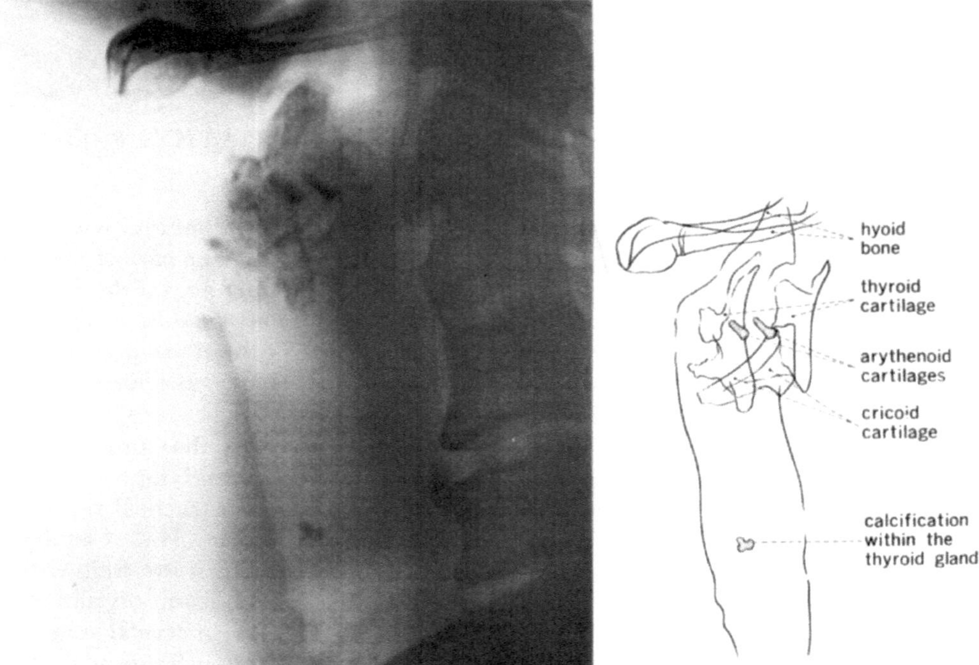

Fig. 34 b   Lateral view of the female neck to show the ossifying process occurring in the posterior parts of the thyroid cartilage, in the plate and the postero-lateral aspect of the arch of the cricoid cartilage. The ossified arythenoid cartilages are seen as dense shadows.   The patient is a fifty-one year-old female.

LARYNGO-TRACHEAL AIR COLUMN AND ESOPHAGUS

The airway is clearly outlined on lateral roentgenograms because of its low radiological density. When a sagittal view is obtained, the higher kilovoltage provides better visualization of the air column. Displacement, compression, indentation and invasion of the trachea must be carefully studied. These signs are produced from either side, from in front, or from behind by the enlarged thyroid nodules. It must be stressed that, before a diagnosis of malignancy can be made, there must be clear evidence of invasion, not merely displacement or indentation. Invasion of the trachea is best demonstrated on tomograms. In cases where there are signs and symptoms suggesting the presence of esophageal invasion, examination by barium swallow is also indicated.

Chapter VI

Clinical Application and Results

Since January 1, 1970, soft tissue roentgenography of the neck has been applied as one of the routine examinations for patients with clinical evidence of nodular disorders of the thyroid. The experience with this technique during the 23-month period until November 30, 1971 indicates that it is a promising method for detecting thyroid carcinoma.

INDICATIONS FOR SOFT TISSUE ROENTGENOGRAPHY OF THE THYROID

The main purpose of thyroid soft tissue roentgenography lies first in a detection of thyroid nodules containing calcific deposits and secondly in differentiation between the benign and malignant nodules.

Soft tissue roentgenography may be applied to all the patients with thyroid disease, but some selection of patients for this examination would be preferable in order to avoid unnecessary x-ray exposure. In our series, the examination was performed in all patients with apparent thyroid nodules or with signs and symptoms indicating the possibility of occult carcinoma of the thyroid, such as recurrent nerve palsy of obscure cause, or metastatic lesion of the lung or bone without a known primary tumor.

In patients with known toxic or nontoxic diffuse goiter and those with known subacute or chronic thyroiditis, roentgenograms of the neck were taken during the early stages of this study. It soon became apparent, however, that no calcification was present in thyroid glands affected by these diseases. Thereafter, roentgenograms were taken only when there was evidence of a nodular disorder in addition to the primary disease.

The selection of patients for roentgenography of the neck was performed by one of the authors (Y. F.) based on the routine physical and laboratory examinations. He has been working in the field of thyroid lesions for more than 15 years and has experienced a great variety of signs and symptoms of thyroid cancer. For those physicians who have less experience, it is recommended to extend indications for soft tissue roentgenography over those patients whose primary lesions are thought to be Graves' disease or chronic thyroidits, because thyroid cancer occasionally occurs in association with those thyroid diseases and in such cases the cancer nodule is usually difficult to palpate, and also some of the thyroid cancers appear as a diffusely enlarged, firm goiter so that they simulate chronic thyroiditis on physical examination. In those cases, one lateral soft tissue roentgenogram seems to be sufficient as the routine examination of intrathyroidal calcification.

PATIENTS AND METHODS

During the 23-month period from January 1, 1970 through November 30, 1971, soft tissue roentgenograms of the neck were obtained in a total of 249 patients, of whom 125 were operated upon or biopsied. In each case, one lateral and one or more spot-tangential views were taken.

In 114 patients, most of whom visited the hospital in the first year of the present study, a standard lateral roentgenogram of the neck was also taken for comparison with soft tissue roentgenograms as to detectability of intrathyroidal calcification. The equipment generally used in diagnostic roentgenography was utilized. The exposure factors were: 150 cm target-to-film distance, 72 kVp, 200 mA, and 0.12 sec. The medical x-ray film was used with intensifying screen type FS and Bucky diaphragm 5:1, and automatic processing was used.

After operation, roentgenograms of the surgically removed specimens were obtained in most cases of carcinoma and occasional cases with benign lesions, using soft tissue technique.

COMPARISON OF THREE TYPES OF NECK ROENTGENOGRAMS

The three types of roentgenograms of the neck were available in 114 patients. In each patient, the standard lateral view, the lateral soft tissue roentgenogram and the spot-tangential soft tissue roentgenograms were retrospectively reviewed in that order.

Table 7 Intrathyroidal Calcifications Identified on Three Types of Roentgenograms of the Neck.

Type of Roentgenogram	No. of patients examined	Calcification on roentgenogram			
		None	Coarse alone	Psammo-matous alone	Combined
Lateral projection, standard roentgenogram	114	83	29	2	0
Lateral projection, soft tissue roentgenogram	114	69	41	3	1
Spot-tangential projection, soft tissue roentgenogram	114	67	39	5	3

The results are shown in Table 7. The standard roentgenograms showed psammomatous shadows in two instances, both of which proved to have papillary carcinoma of the thyroid containing multiple psammoma bodies in conglomerated form. Coarse calcifications were observed in 29 cases. The lateral soft tissue roentgenograms revealed much better defined coarse calcific deposits than shown on the standard roentgenograms, and an additional 13 more cases were found to contain coarse deposits. However, as far as psammomatous calcifications were concerned, only two more cases were detected by this technique. The spot-tangential views obtained by our newly developed technique gave far better results in the detection of psammomatous calcification; combined psammomatous and coarse calcifications were observed in three instances and psammomatous alone in five. All the eight patients who were positive for psammomatous calcifications proved to have thyroid cancers and thus there were no false positives in this series.

Although the lateral projection with soft tissue technique did not always present satisfactory results in the detection of psammomatous calcifications, it proved to be as good or slightly superior to the spot-tangential views for the visualization of coarse calcifications, because the lateral view provided sufficient detail to clearly identify the coarse calcifications with the same reliability as the spot-tangential view and had the advantage of presenting a wider field, so that the localization of the calcified area became easier, and occasionally, as we experienced in case 14 (Chapter 7, p. 103), calcified nodules located in unexpected sites were incidentally found.

CALCIFICATIONS ON SOFT TISSUE ROENTGENOGRAMS OF THE NECK

The results of roentgenologic examination of intrathyroidal calcifications in a total of 249 patients are shown in Tables 8 and 9, divided according to the histologically proven and unproven cases, respectively.

In the patients presented in Table 8, radical operation was carried out in all of the 52 patients with malignant tumors of the thyroid except for two; one with anaplastic carcinoma and one with malignant lymphoma. The former was treated with irradiation after biopsy and in the latter partial resection was followed by irradiation. The 42 patients with adenomas and 14 patients with adenomatous goiters were treated surgically with removal of the nodules and one patient with Graves' disease underwent a subtotal thyroidectomy. The diagnosis of chronic thyroiditis was confirmed in 15 instances by needle biopsy and one case of subacute thyroiditis by open biopsy.

Table 8   Calcifications on Roentgenograms of the Neck in Patients with Histologically Proven Lesions.

Pathological classification	Total No. of patients	Calcification on roentgenogram			
		None	Coarse alone	Psammo-matous alone	Combined
Thyroid cancer	52	12	27	9	4
Thyroid adenoma	42	28	14	0	0
Adenomatous goiter	14	2	12	0	0
Chronic thyroiditis*	15	15	0	0	0
Subacute thyroiditis**	1	1	0	0	0
Graves' disease	1	1	0	0	0
Total	125	59	53	9	4

 * Diagnoses were confirmed by needle biopsies.
** Diagnosis was confirmed by open biopsy. This was an unusual case, in which subacute granulomatous thyroiditis tecurred 10 years after the first attack.

It is worth mentioning that, of these histologically proven 125 cases, the thirteen that showed either psammomatous calcification alone or combined psammomatous and coarse calcifications all proved to have thyroid cancer. No false positive cases were found. Thus the presence of psammomatous calcification on preoperative roentgenograms of the neck can be considered as diagnostic of carcinoma. In the 52 cases of thyroid cancer, the incidence of psammomatous calcifications found on the roentgenograms was 25 per cent and this low percentage reflects the difficulty of demonstrating psammoma bodies even with the special methods applied in this study. Microscopic examination revealed the presence of psammoma bodies in 26 of these 52 cancers, or 50 per cent (Table 11).

Coarse calcifications were found on the roentgenograms of the neck in 31 of 52 cancers, or 60 per cent, in 14 of 42 adenomas, or 34 per cent, and in 12 of 14 adenomatous goiters, or 86 per cent. The correlation of the variety of coarse calcifications with the histologic diagnoses will be discussed later (p. 62, (3)).

The incidence of calcifications in patients whose thyroid lesions are as yet not histologically proven is presented in Table 9. The diagnostic impressions were derived from the physical and laboratory findings, thyroid scintigram and ultrasonic scanning. The diagnosis of cancer in eight instances were almost conclusive from their history of palliative operations in the past or physical findings of a hard, fixed nodule associated with lymph node swelling, or a demonstration of psammomatous calcifications on neck roentgenograms. Those nodules classified as adenomas were mostly single nodules with benign appearance on the physical examination and more than half of them proved to be "cystic" by ultrasound scanning. In these cases, percutaneous puncture with aspiration of the cyst fluid was performed. The diagnostic impression of adenomatous goiter was based mainly on the physical findings and most of these patients had a long history of goiter.

Table 9 Calcifications on Roentgenograms of the Neck in Patients with Histologically Unproven Lesions.

Clinical diagnosis	Total No. of patients	Calcification on roentgenogram			
		None	Coarse alone	Psammomatous alone	Combined
Thyroid cancer	8	1	5	1	1
Thyroid adenoma	66	54	12	0	0
Adenomatous goiter	21	10	11	0	0
Miscellaneous	29	25	4	0	0
Total	124	90	32	1	1

Of course, it could not be ruled out that a few cases of cancer might be included in those classified as adenoma or adenomatous goiter.

In the histologically unproven series shown in Table 9, there were one patient who was positive for psammomatous calcification alone and another patient who had combined psammomatous and coarse calcifications, for whom operation is being considered with a strong suspicion of cancer. Coarse calcium deposits were found in 6 of 8 patients who probably have thyroid cancers. The incidence of coarse deposits in patients with probable adenoma and adenomatous goiter was 18 per cent and 52 per cent, respectively, the ratios being far less than those found in the histologically proven series. One of the reasons appears to be that, in the unproven adenoma group, more than half of the nodules were thought to be colloid adenomas which had undergone cystic degeneration and most of them had an episode of bleeding within the nodule, and this type of case is usually negative for calcification.

At the present time it is our policy not to perform surgery for a symptomless adenomatous goiter, unless it presents any sign of thyroid carcinoma, the evidence of which has thus far been obtained by detection of small, irregular, hard nodules by careful palpation or by the demonstration of small, coarse, dense calcifications on roentgenograms of the neck. The fact that the incidence of coarse calcification was high in the proven adenomatous goiters and low in the unproven cases may reflect our policy stated above.

ROENTGENOGRAPHIC FINDINGS IN PATIENTS WITH THYROID CANCER

1. Comparison Between Lateral and Spot-Tangential Soft Tissue Roentgenograms

Here again we wish to compare the results obtained by lateral views of the neck with those obtained by spot-tangential views in the cancer patients. As shown in Table 10,

Table 10 Calcifications on Lateral Views and Spot-Tangential Views of Soft-Tissue Roentgenography in Sixty Patients with Proven and Unproven Thyroid Cancers.

Projection	Total No. of patients	Calcification on roentgenogram			
		None	Coarse alone	Psammomatous alone	Combined
Lateral view	60	27	35	7	1
Spot-tangential view	60	13	32	10	5

it is apparent that for the demonstration of psammomatous calcifications the spot-tangential view is far superior to the lateral view. This was especially true when the psammoma bodies were non-conglomerated or not numerous. In reading of the roentgenograms, identification of psammomatous calcification was easier if a high intensity light was used, rather than the usual method of placing the films on a conventional view box.

2. Correlation Between Findings on Neck Roentgenogram, Specimen Roentgenogram and Histologic Sections

The calcifications observed on the preoperative soft tissue roentgenograms of the neck were correlated with those on the specimen roentgenograms and the histologic sections. As shown in Table 11, all 13 cases that presented psammomatous calcifications on the neck roentgenograms also showed positive shadows on the specimen roentgenograms.

Table 11 Calcifications on Roentgenograms of Neck, Specimen Roentgenograms

Patient	Histology of cancer	Roentgenogram of neck Ps*	Roentgenogram of neck Co**	Specimen roentgenogram Ps*	Specimen roentgenogram Co**	Histologic section Ps*	Histologic section Co**
1. WA 35 F	Papillary	+	+	not available		+	+
2. OK 43 F	Papillary	+	+	+	+	+	+
3. HN 52 F	Papillary	+	+	+	+	+	+
4. AI 56 F	Follicular	+	+	+	+	+	+
5. IM 45 F	Papillary	+	−	+	−	+	−
6. NO 26 F	Papillary	+	−	+	−	+	−
7. KT 23 F	Papillary	+	−	+	−	+	−
8. TN 28 M	Papillary	+	−	+	−	+	−
9. MS 29 M	Papillary	+	−	+	−	+	−
10. AY 26 M	Papillary	+	−	+	−	+	−
11. ST 14 F	Papillary	+	−	+	−	+	−
12. TB 10 F	Papillary	+	−	+	−	+	−
13. HT 59 F	Papillary	+	−	+	−	+	−
14. SY 63 M	Papillary	−	+	−	+	+	+
15. AM 49 F	Papillary	−	+	−	+	−	+
16. NB 50 F	Papillary	−	+	not available		−	+
17. KJ 37 F	Papillary	−	+	+	+	+	+
18. OZ 54 F	Papillary	−	+	+	+	+	+
19. KT 40 F	Papillary	−	+	−	+	+	+
20. KY 40 F	Papillary	−	+	not available		+	+
21. SY 56 F	Papillary	−	+	−	+	−	+
22. AP 42 F	Papillary	−	+	−	+	+	+
23. YG 59 F	Papillary	−	+	−	+	−	+
24. SM 77 F	Papillary	−	+	not available		−	+
25. HT 49 M	Follicular	−	+	not available		−	+
26. IU 40 F	Papillary	−	+	−	+	−	+

* Ps: Psammomatous calcification on roentgenograms, or psammoma bodies in histologic sections.

The presence of psammoma bodies was also confirmed on the histologic sections.

The other 39 cases did not show psammomatous calcifications on the neck roentgenograms, but 13 cases, or a third of them, actually had psammoma bodies in the histologic sections. In 10 of these 13 cases, specimen roentgenograms were obtained, and psammomatous calcifications were definitely identified in only two of them. The psammoma bodies demonstrated only on histologic examinations were usually nonconglomerated, scattered and were in numbers of less than 10 in one histologic section. These carcinomas contained too few psammoma bodies to be demonstrated even on the most technically optimal roentgenograms now available. If a more refined roentgenographic technique were available, psammomatous calcifications could probably be identified in a few more instances where psammoma bodies were already present in enough number for their demonstration on specimen roentgenograms.

and Histologic Sections in 52 Patients with Histologically Proven Thyroid Cancers.

Patient	Histology of cancer	Roentgenogram of neck		Specimen roentgenogram		Histologic section	
		Ps*	Co**	Ps*	Co**	Ps*	Co**
27. ST 40 F	Papillary	—	+	not available		—	+
28. TD 61 F	Papillary	—	+	—	+	—	+
29. SK 61 M	Papillary	—	+	—	+	+	+
30. HZ 45 F	Papillary	—	+	—	+	—	+
31. ST 32 F	Papillary	—	+	not available		—	+
32. NI 44 M	Follicular	—	+	—	+	—	+
33. NG 52 F	Follicular	—	+	—	+	—	+
34. HT 49 M	Follicular	—	+	not available		—	+
35. ID 28 F	Follicular	—	+	not available		—	+
36. KS 23 F	Papillary	—	+	not available		+	+
37. TG 50 F	Papillary	—	+	—	+	+	+
38. TZ 62 F	Follicular	—	+	—	+	—	+
39. TD 48 F	Follicular	—	+	—	+	—	+
40. KT 39 F	Papillary	—	+	—	+	—	+
41. KS 38 M	Follicular	—	—	—	—	—	—
42. GT 46 M	Medullary	—	—	—	—	—	—
43. KS 29 F	Papillary	—	—	not available		+	—
44. TK 48 M	Papillary	—	—	—	—	—	—
45. TB 68 F	Anaplastic	—	—	not available		—	—
46. ND 33 F	Papillary	—	—	not available		+	—
47. AK 35 F	Papillary	—	—	—	—	+	—
48. MD 24 F	Papillary	—	—	—	—	—	—
49. MZ 64 F	Lymphoma	—	—	not available		—	—
50. NM 72 M	Follicular	—	—	not available		—	—
51. MS 20 F	Follicular	—	—	—	—	—	—
52. MT 25 F	Papillary	—	—	—	—	+	—

** Co: Coarse calcific deposit on roentgenograms, or coarse and amorphous calcific deposit in histologic sections.

3. Calcifications on Soft Tissue Roentgenogram in Relation to Thyroid Cancer Histology

Calcifications identified on soft tissue roentgenograms of the neck were correlated with the histological classification in cases of thyroid cancer. As shown in Table 12, of the 13 cases that were positive for psammomatous calcification, 12 or 92 per cent were papillary carcinoma and only one was follicular carcinoma. On the other hand, coarse calcifications were found in 23 or 61 per cent of 38 papillary carcinomas and 8 or 73 per cent of 11 follicular carcinomas.

Table 12 Calcifications on Roentgenograms of the Neck in Relation to Thyroid Cancer Histology.

Pathological classification	Total No. of patients	Calcification on roentgenogram			
		None	Coarse alone	Psammo-matous alone	Combined
Papillary carcinoma	38	6	20	9	3
Follicular carcinoma	11	3	7	0	1
Medullary carcinoma with amyloid stroma	1	1	0	0	0
Anaplastic carcinoma	1	1	0	0	0
Malignant lymphoma	1	1	0	0	0
Total	52	12	27	9	4

In marked contrast to these differentiated carcinomas, which tend to grow slowly and have a relatively good prognosis, no calcium deposits were found in the cancers with more aggressive growth, such as medullary and anaplastic carcinomas and the one case of malignant lymphoma.

4. Correlation of Physical Findings with Radiological Evidence of Calcification

When the physical findings are correlated with roentgenologic evidence of calcifications in the patients with thyroid cancer, the diagnostic value of the soft tissue roentgenograms of the neck becomes more apparent. The 52 histologically proven cases of thyroid cancer and the 8 unquestionable but as yet unproven cases of thyroid cancer were divided according to physical findings into the following seven groups:

Group I: Diagnostic impression of cancer of the thyroid was obtained at physical examination, because of the presence of a hard, irregular, fixed nodule of the thyroid and clinically apparent lymph node metastases (T3, N1, 2 or 3, as classified according to TNM Classification).

Group II: Diagnostic impression at physical examination was probable cancer, because of the presence of a hard, fixed, irregular thyroid nodule but without clinical evidence of lymph node metastases (T3, N 0).

Group III: Those having enlarged lymph nodes in the neck without a palpable primary lesion in the thyroid gland. Most of these cases had biopsies of the involved lymph nodes and were proven histologically to be metastatic thyroid carcinoma (T0, N1, 2 or 3).

Group IV: A round, freely movable thyroid nodule of varying size. Clinically a benign nodule was suspected.

Group V: In association with a clinically apparent benign nodule, a small carcinoma was incidentally found during a careful preoperative examination, during the operation or at the histological examination. Clinically only the benign nodule was evident and the small carcinoma was not detectable or often overlooked.

Group VI: Special type of papillary carcinoma which was characterized by diffuse thyroid infiltration and association with an autoimmune thyroiditis. Clinically the thyroid gland was diffusely enlarged, firm, and the disease simulated chronic thyroiditis on physical and laboratory examinations.

Group VII: Thyroid cancer occurred within the diffusely enlarged thyroid gland affected by either Graves' disease or chronic thyroiditis. It was not necessarily easy to palpate the cancer nodule preoperatively.

Three important conclusions can be drawn from this correlative study between physical findings and roentgenographic demonstration of either psammomatous or coarse calcification (Table 13).

(1) Of the 15 cases that were positive for psammomatous calcifications on the roentgenograms of the neck, 11 had the physical findings classified as Group III, IV, VI or VII. Thus, psammomatous calcifications which can be considered as definitive indication of the presence of thyroid cancer were found mostly in those patients who were difficult to diagnose as having cancer by the physical examination as well as by other laboratory studies.

During the period of the present study, we found two special types of papillary carcinoma, in which only the roentgenographic demonstration of psammomatous calcification could provide a definitive diagnostic clue as to the presence of malignancy.

One of them is represented by three patients in Group IV. The cancer appeared as a round, movable nodule of 3 to 6 cm in diameter and simulated a benign adenoma on the physical examination. They were all well-encapsulated papillary carcinomas with histological evidence of minimal invasion and contained numerous psammoma bodies. All three patients were young males who were 26, 28 and 29 years old.

The other type of papillary carcinoma was classified above in Group VI, and had in many respects the opposite characteristics of the type mentioned above. Namely, the two patients were both girls whose ages were 10 and 14, and the gross and microscopic examinations revealed a marked intrathyroidal infiltration of cancer cells.

(2) The cases in Group I and II were readily diagnosed as thyroid cancer on physical examination. The radiological evidence of psammoma bodies was obtained in only four of the 35 cases. The more important fact is that 23 cases presented coarse calcifications and all of the 15 histologically proven cases among them were those with well-differentiated papillary or follicular carcinomas. Of the 10 proven cases that were negative for any form of calcification on roentgenograms of the neck, five or 50 per cent were poorly differentiated carcinomas such as solid variant of follicular carcinoma, anaplastic carcinoma, or malignant lymphoma. These results imply that, if the coarse calcifications are found on roentgenograms of the neck in patients with clinically apparent carcinomas, it may indicate the presence of chronic pathologic processes such as a densely fibrous capsule or massive fibrosis within or around the tumor and the lesions are usually slow growing differentiated carcinomas. On the other hand, the absence of the radiologic evidence of calcium deposits in the thyroid harboring clinically apparent cancers often indicates the presence of a rapidly growing, less differentiated malignant neoplasm. Here we have to mention that not rarely an anaplastic carcinoma may arise from a well differentiated thyroid carcinoma having radiological evidence of calcification.

Table 13 Correlation of Physical Findings

Group*: Physical findings		Total number of patients
I	A firm or hard, irregular, fixed nodule of the thyroid with palpable lymph nodes in the neck.	9
II	A firm or hard, irregular, fixed nodule of the thyroid without palpable lymph nodes in the neck.	26
III	Enlarged lymph nodes in the neck without an easily palpable primary lesion in the thyroid.	5
IV	A round, movable nodule of the thyroid, size variable. No palpable lymph nodes.	11
V	Incidentally found small carcinoma in association with clinically apparent benign thyroid nodule(s).	1
VI	Diffusely enlarged, firm goiter with or without palpable lymph nodes in the neck (Diffusely infiltrating papillary carcinoma)	3
VII	Palpable or non-palpable cancer nodule within a diffuse goiter of Graves' disease or of chronic thyroiditis.	5
Total		60

* Ca: Carcinoma, Ad: Adenoma or benign nodule
Papillary: Papillary carcinoma, Follicular: Follicular carcinoma
Follicular solid: Solid variant of follicular carcinoma

In such a case, localization of calcified area within the palpable thyroid nodule is important. The part of recent progressive growth lacks in calcific deposits.

(3) Finally we must mention the diagnostic importance of the coarse calcifications found in the cases of Group III, IV and VII. Coarse calcific deposits, concentrically present in an area less than 1 cm in diameter, usually indicate the presence of occult carcinoma of the thyroid. In fact, the above statement was evidenced in the four patients of Group VII, who had small carcinomas within diffuse goiters, and in the three patients of Group III who presented recurrent nerve palsy or lymph node metastasis with un-

with Radiological Evidence of Calcification.

Calcification on roentgenograms of the neck			
Psammomatous and coarse	Psammomatous alone	Coarse alone	None
1 (Papillary 1)		5 (Papillary 3 / ? 2)	3 (Papillary 1 / Follicular solid 1 / Medullary 1)
2 (Papillary 1 / ? 1)	1 (Papillary 1)	15 (Papillary 11 / Follicular 1 / ? 3)	8 (Papillary 4 / Follicular solid 1 / Anaplastic 1 / Lymphoma 1 / ? 1)
	2 (Occult papillary 2)	3 (Occult papillary 3)	
1 (Follicular 1)	5 (Papillary 4 / ? 1)	5 (Papillary 1 / Follicular 3 / Occult follicular 1)	
			1 (Occult follicular 1)
	2 (Papillary 2)		1 (Occult papillary 1)
1 (Papillary 1)		4 (Occult papillary 2 / Follicular 1 / Occult follicular 1)	
5	10	32	13

Medullary: Medullary carcinoma (solid carcinoma with amyloid stroma)
Anaplastic: Anaplastic carcinoma, Lymphoma: Malignant lymphoma of the thyroid
?: Case not yet operated, Occult: carcinoma less than 1.5 cm in diameter.

known primary. One of the patients in Group IV was a 52-year-old woman who had had a metastatic lesion in the frontal bone for two years and was referred to us for a search of the primary lesion. Although the thyroid scintigram did not show a cold nodule, a small nodule approximately 1 cm in diameter was palpated in the right lobe of the thyroid and roentgenograms of the neck revealed a round calcific deposit. The nodule was removed and histologically disclosed to be the primary lesion of follicular carcinoma of the thyroid. Thus by revealing evidence of calcified nodules, roentgenograms of the neck provide a means of identifying and localizing small carcinomas that are, otherwise, not clinically detectable.

Chapter VII

Case Reports

Because the clinical appearances of both benign and malignant thyroid nodules vary greatly, it will be very helpful for the reader to review as many cases with different physical findings as possible.

Case reports are arranged in the following three categories:

(1) Carcinoma of the thyroid that presented psammomatous calcification alone or in association with coarse calcific deposits on soft tissue roentgenograms of the neck preoperatively (Case 1-9).

(2) Carcinoma of the thyroid that presented coarse calcification alone on the neck films preoperatively (Case 10-18).

(3) Benign nodules of the thyroid that showed coarse calcification on the neck films preoperatively (Case 19-24).

I. CARCINOMA OF THE THYROID PRESENTING PSAMMOMATOUS CALCIFICATION ON THE NECK FILMS

A. Diffusely Infiltrative Type of Papillary Carcinoma of the Thyroid (Case 1, 2)

This type is classified as Group VI in Table 13.

The type of papillary carcinoma of the thyroid presented here is difficult to diagnose by routine physical and laboratory examinations, but soft tissue roentgenography of the neck provides a valuable diagnostic clue. The disease is characterized by a diffuse infiltration of cancer cells involving the entire or almost the entire thyroid gland and is consistantly accompanied by an autoimmune thyroiditis. The thyroid gland is usually firm and diffusely enlarged and may simulate Hashimoto's disease.

This particular type of papillary carcinoma is seen almost exclusively in young females. A descrete cold nodule on the thyroid scintigram, if observed, is indicative of the presence of a neoplasm in the thyroid affected by chronic thyroiditis. The primary tumor is, however, large enough to present as a cold nodule in less than one half of the patients. Histological examination showed that, in all the cases encountered thus far, numerous psammoma bodies were present in the diffusely infiltrating cancer cell masses. It is expected that detection of psammomatous calcification on the soft tissue roentgenogram of the neck would be very useful in diagnosing this unique type of thyroid cancer. It, in fact, proved to be true in the two cases whose histories follow.

Case 1. A Diffuse Goiter of Firm Consistency Seen in a Girl: Diffusely Infiltrating Papillary Carcinoma

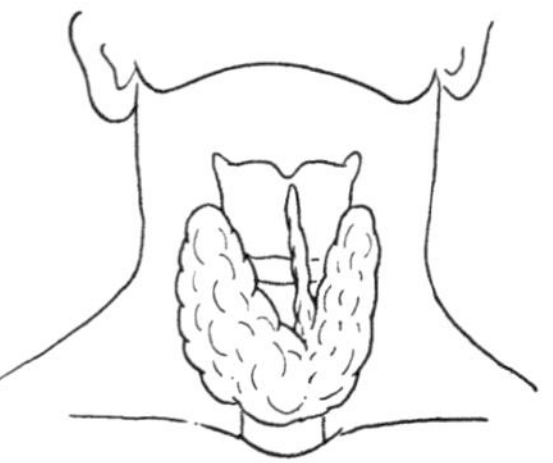

Fig. 35

S. T., a 14-year-old girl first noticed thyroid swelling in February, 1970. Subacute thyroiditis was suspected because of the firm enlargement of the right lobe with slight tenderness and an increased erythrocyte sedimentation rate (ESR) of 43 mm per hour. Prednisone was administered. Two months later, the patient was referred to us for further evaluation, because the symptoms did not respond well to steroid therapy.

Examination revealed a diffusely enlarged thyroid, measuring 2.5×6 cm on the right and 1.5×5 cm on the left (Fig. 35). It was firm, non-tender and fixed to the trachea. No cervical lymph nodes were palpable. ^{131}I thyroid uptake at 24 hours was 23.3% and T_3 resin sponge uptake (RSU) was 22.4%. Thyroid scintigram was interpreted as normal (Fig. 36). The tanned red cell hemagglutination test (TRC) was positive at 1: 10^6 dilution, but anti-microsomal antibody was negative by the indirect immunofluorescent antibody technique. ESR was 31 mm per hour.

Autoimmune thyroiditis was suspected and to confirm the diagnosis a needle biopsy was performed. Sections revealed lymphocytic infiltration with an aggregate of psammoma bodies (Fig. 37), which was indicative of the presence of papillary carcinoma of the thyroid. Then soft tissue roentgenograms of the neck showed numerous minute calcific shadows typical of psammoma bodies. (Fig. 38).

At operation, the thyroid was diffusely enlarged and multiple metastases were found in cervical lymph nodes bilaterally. Total thyroidectomy was carried out along with bilateral neck dissections (Figs. 39, 40). The primary lesion located in the center of the right lobe, and invaded locally into the trachea. The superficial cartilage layer of the trachea was removed with the tumor.

The roentgenogram of the surgically removed specimen showed the presence of psammoma bodies distributed throughout the thyroid gland, and also within the paratracheal and jugular lymph nodes (Fig. 41). The permanent paraffin sections revealed that the primary carcinoma was 1 cm in diameter, and the cancer cells were infiltrating via the interlobular lymphatic channels throughout the thyroid gland (Fig. 42). Marked lymphoid cell infiltration associated with lymph follicles having germinal centers were observed in the thyroid parenchyma.

The postperative course was uneventful, and she has been doing well with desiccated thyroid medication.

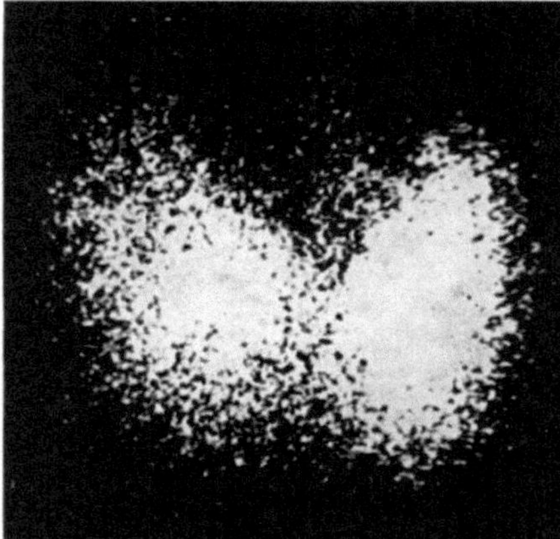

Fig. 36 Thyroid scintigram. The uptake of radioiodine is less in the right lobe than the left, but no apparent cold nodule is present.

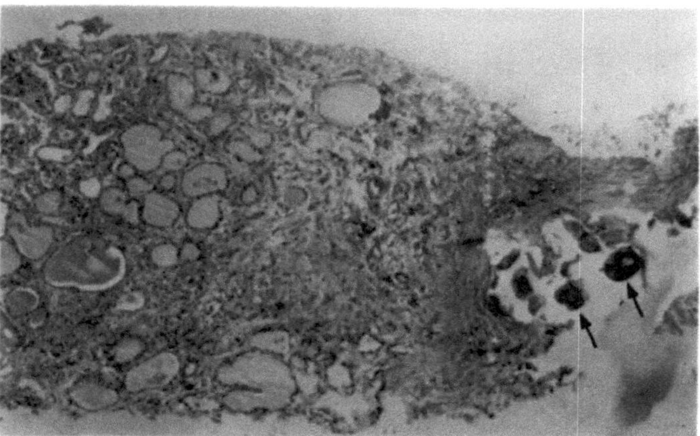

Fig. 37 Microscopic section from a needle biopsy specimen showing inflammatory cell infiltration in the thyroid tissue and aggregates of psammoma bodies (arrows). (H & E. ×60)

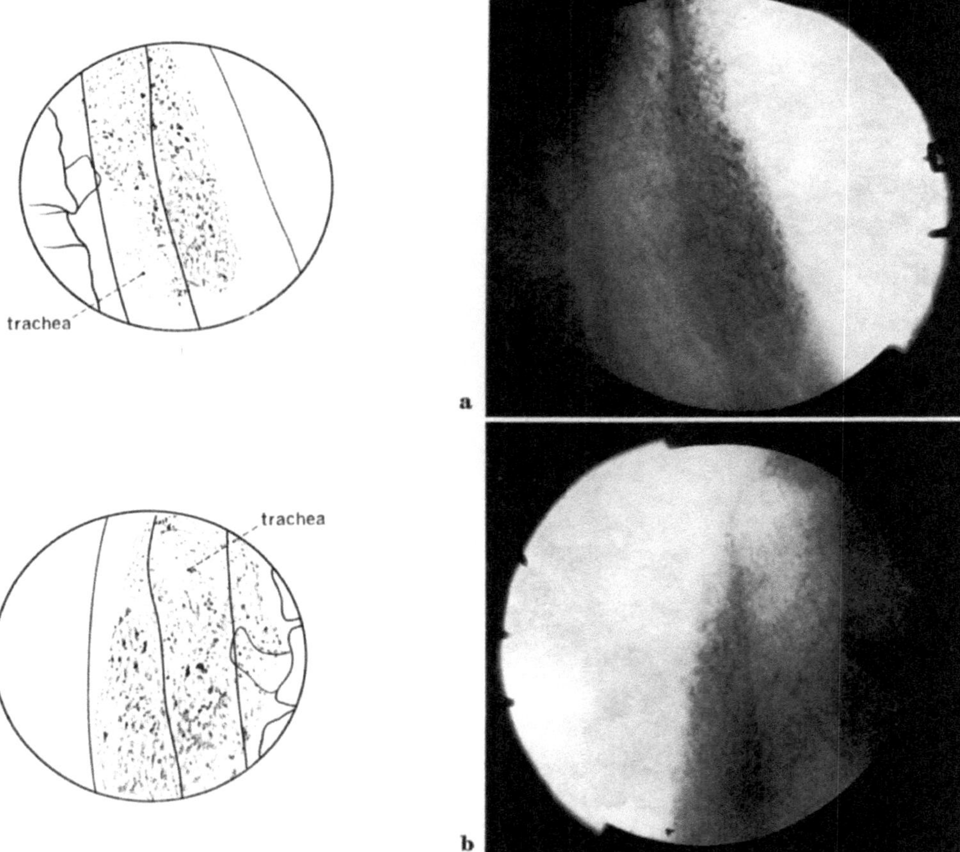

Fig. 38 Spot-tangential views of soft tissue roentgenography of the neck taken on both sides, showing typical psammomatous pattern of calcification; (a) right side and (b) left side.

 CASE REPORTS

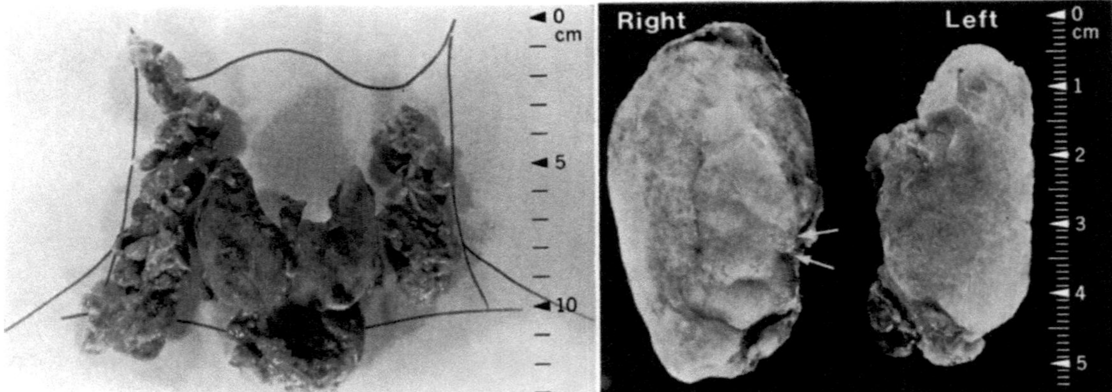

Fig. 39 Resected specimen. Total thyroidectomy and bilateral modified neck dissections were performed.

Fig. 40 Cut surface of the removed thyroid gland. Due to the diffuse infiltration of cancer cells and an associated chronic thyroiditis, the cut surface is homogeneously greyish-yellow and the primary cancer (arrows) is not clearly defined.

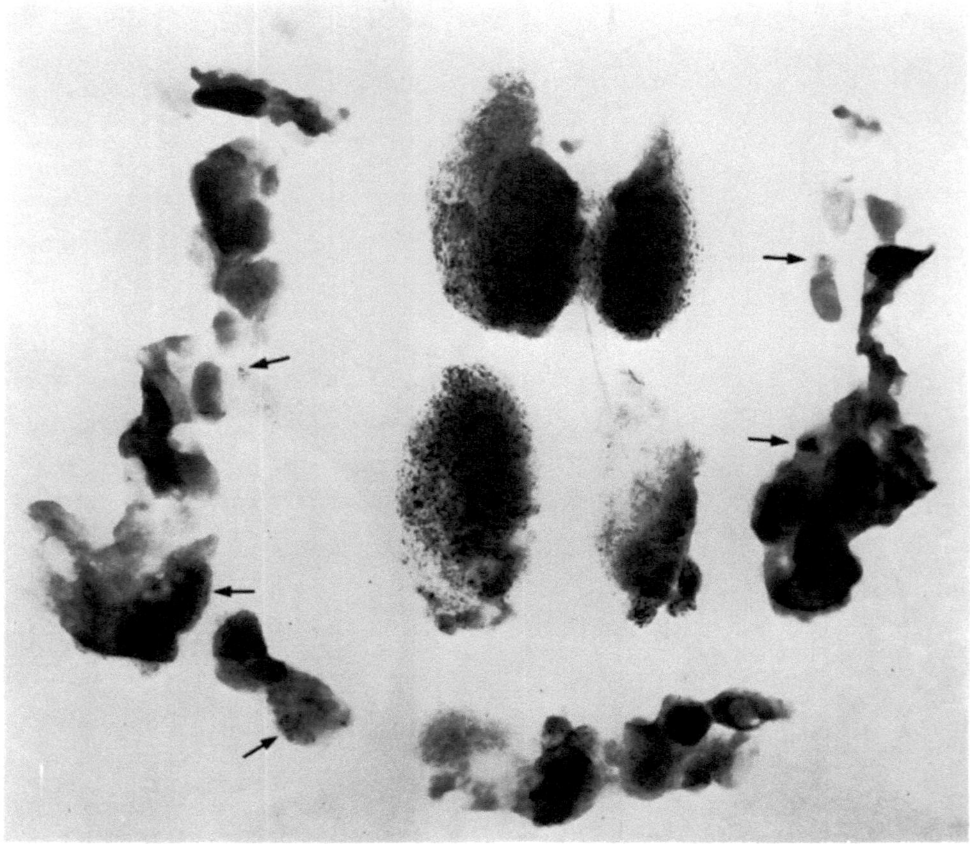

Fig. 41 Roentgenogram of surgica specimen. Note the numerous psammomatous calcifications distributed diffusely throughout the thyroid gland and in the lymph nodes involved by metastatic lesions.

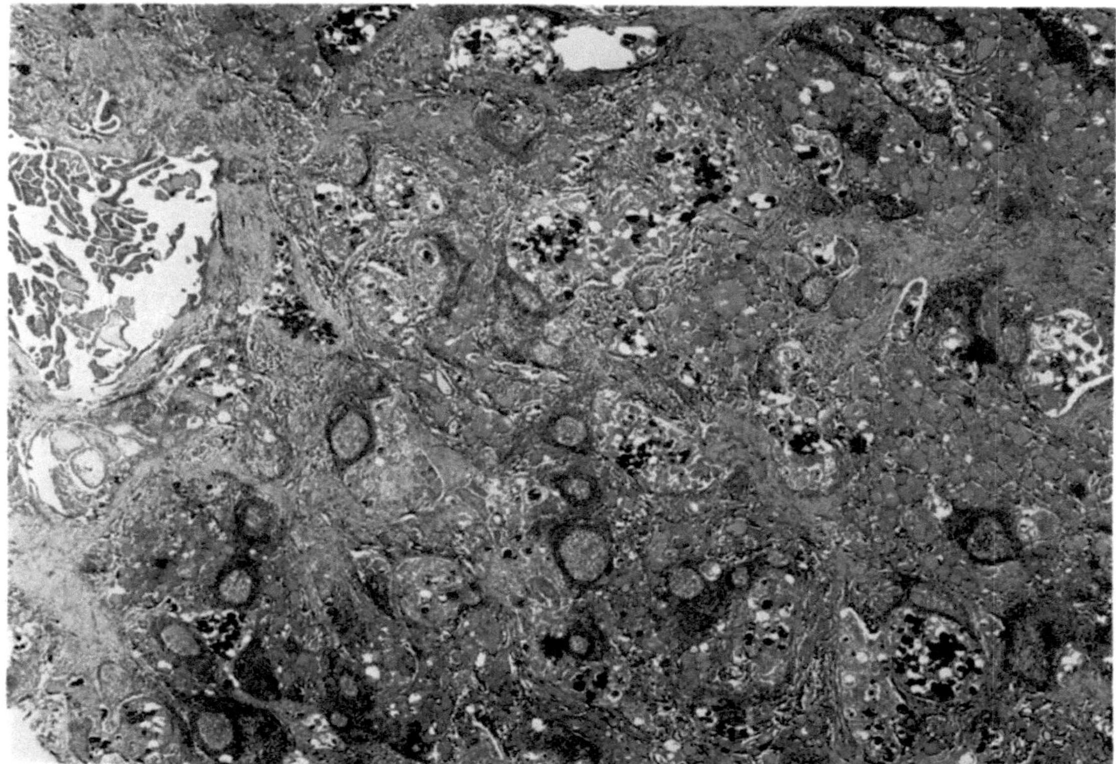

Fig. 42 Low power photomicrograph of the thyroid specimen, showing a papillary growth of the primary cancer lesion in the left upper portion and diffuse intrathyroidal infiltration of cancer cells via interlobular lymphatic channels, where conglomerated psammoma bodies are seen. Lymphoid cell infiltration and lymph-follicle formation are also evident in the thyroid parenchyma. (H & E, ×20)

Case 2.   Another Case of Diffusely Infiltrating Papillary
Carcinoma of the Thyroid

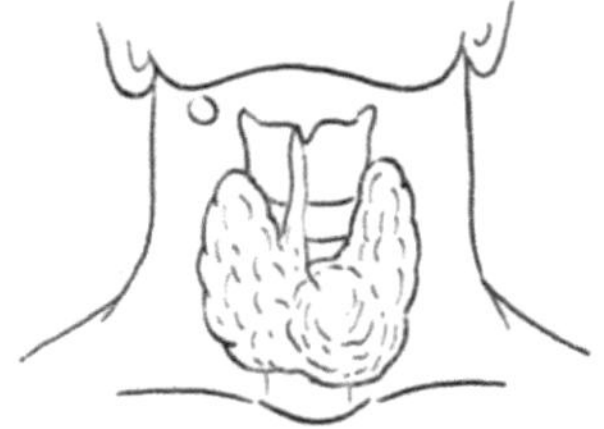

Fig. 43

T. B., a 10-year-old girl visited the hospital in May, 1970, with the chief complaint of
painless swelling of the anterior part of the neck of one month duration.

Examination revealed a diffusely enlarged thyroid measuring 1.5×4 cm on the right
and 2×4.5 cm on the left.   The entire gland was firm, but the area between the left lobe
and the isthmus was particularly hard and slightly irregular (Fig. 43)   A soft, movable
lymph node was palpated in the right submaxillary region.

The T_3 RSU was 24.6%, whereas protein bound iodine was 7.5 μg per 100 ml and
131I uptake was 46.7%, both of which were at the upper limit of, or slightly above the
normal range.   A cold nodule was noted in the lower half of the left lobe and the isthmus
on the scintigram (Fig. 44).   The ESR was 12 mm per hour   Anti-thyroglobulin antibody was detected by TRC test at $1:10^5$ dilution and by the indirect immunofluorescent
antibody technique.

Since this patient was referred to us shortly after we had seen the first case, a suspicion
of diffusely infiltrating papillary carcinoma of the thyroid was entertained, and soft
tissue roentgenograms of the neck revealed psammomatous calcification (Fig. 45).

Total thyroidectomy and bilateral modified neck dissection were performed (Fig. 46).
The roentgenogram of the surgical specimen revealed psammoma bodies distributed
diffusely in the left lobe and isthmus (Fig. 47).   This was confirmed by histological examination (Fig. 48).   The right lobe was affected only by autoimmune thyroiditis.   Lymph
node metastases were found in the paratracheal region bilaterally and in the left jugular
chain.   The right submaxillary lymph node palpated preoperatively proved to be negative
for malignancy.

The postoperative course was smooth except for the development of tetany, which has
been controlled by 3 grams of calcium lactate daily.   She has been doing well for one
year while receiving 75 mg of desiccated thyroid daily.

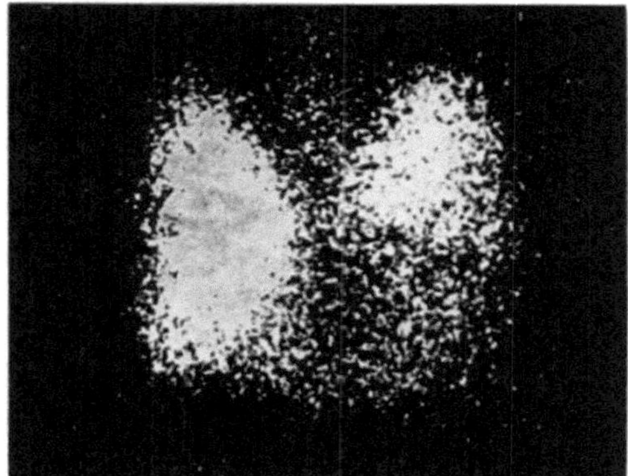

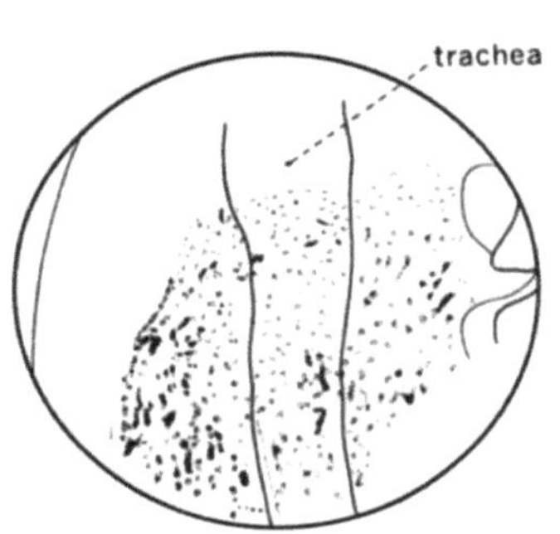

Fig. 44 Thyroid scintigram showing a cold nodule in the lower half of the left lobe.

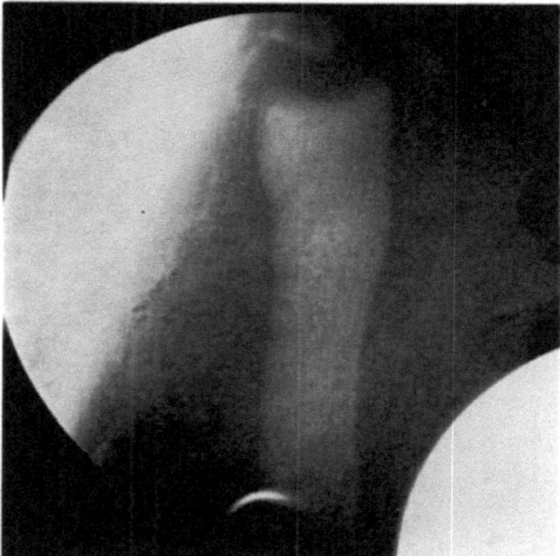

Fig. 45 Spot-tangential view of the neck. Numerous psammomatous calcifications are evident.

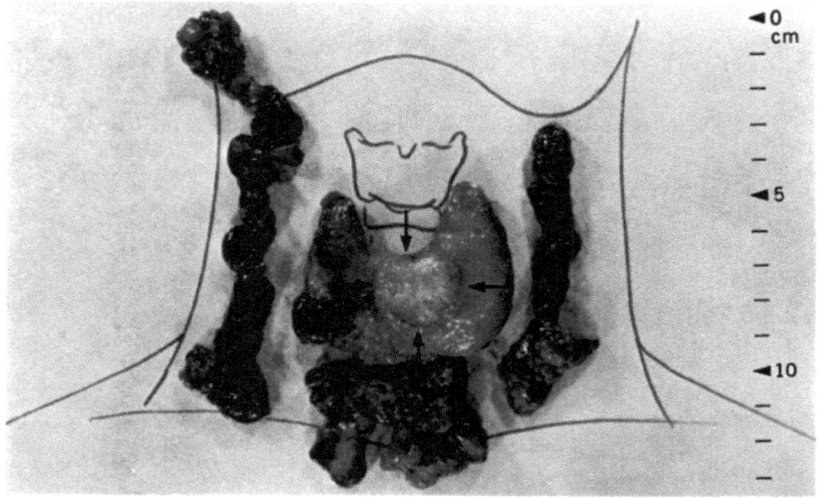

Fig. 46 Surgically removed specimen. Total thyroidectomy and bilateral modified neck dissections were carried out. On a cut surface of the thyroid, the primary lesion (arrows) is clearly seen.

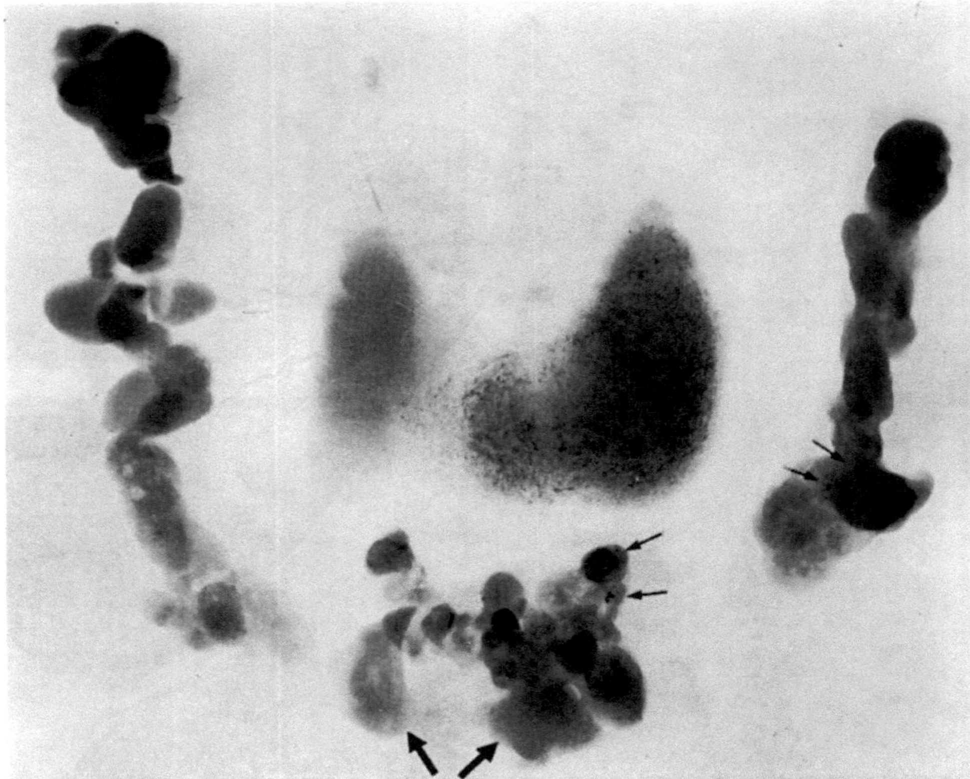

Fig. 47 Specimen roentgenogram. Note numerous psammomatous calcifications are distributed diffusely throughout the left lobe and isthmus, which indicate the extent of intrathyroidal infiltration of cancer cells. Calcified shadows are also evident in the involved lymph nodes (small arrows). Numerous minute calcific deposits seen within the resected thymic tissue (large arrows) represent calcified Hassal's bodies.

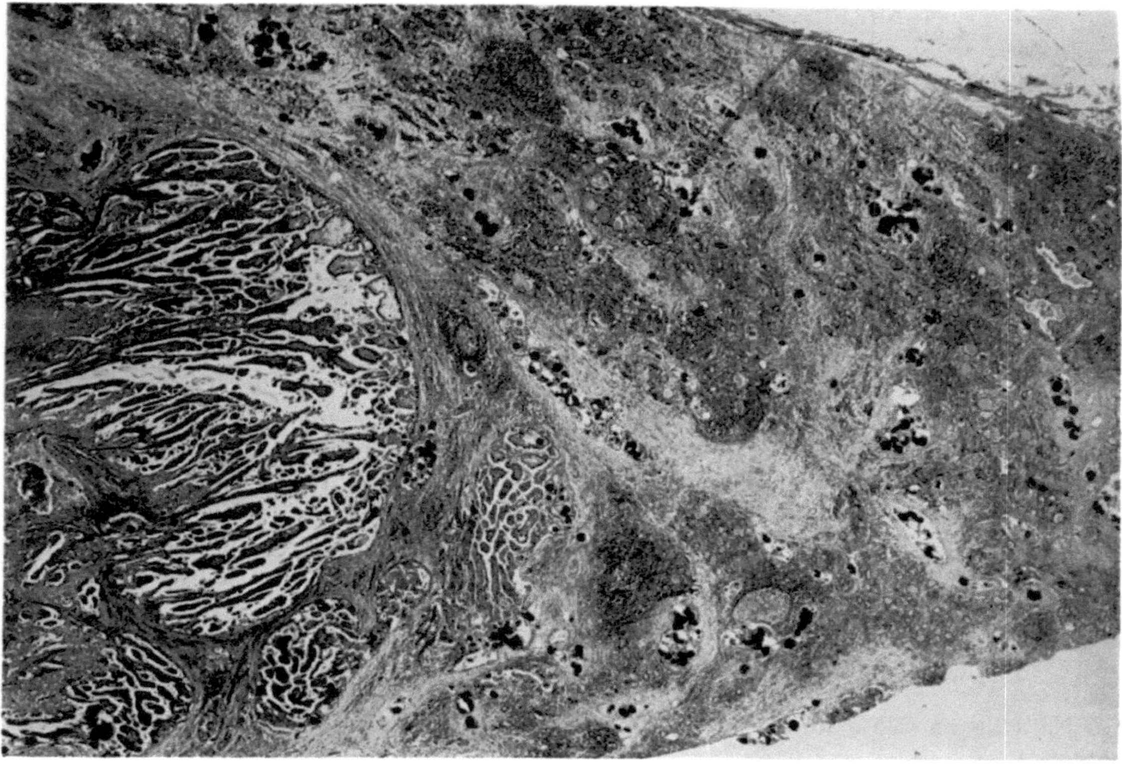

Fig. 48 Photomicrograph of thyroid specimen, showing the primary lesion of papillary carcinoma in the left portion and diffuse intrathyroidal infiltration of cancer cells accompanied by psammoma bodies (seen as black, punctate granules on the photomicrograph). There are also marked inflammatory infiltrate and lymph follicle formation. (H & E, ×10)

B.   Grossly Non-Infiltrative Type of Papillary Carcinoma of the Thyroid
     (Cases 3-5)
This type is classified as Group IV in Table 13.
The following three cases are good examples illustrating the opposite extreme of papillary carcinoma of the thyroid as compared to the aforementioned small primary lesion with diffuse infiltrative growth as seen in Case 1 and 2.   Although two of the lesions are large and one is small in size, all of them are characterized by a well-outlined, round tumor, without palpable lymph nodes in the neck.   Only the psammomatous calcification detected on the neck films provided a definite diagnostic clue.

Case 3.   A Large, Round, Movable Nodule Seen in a
             Young Man: Non-Invasive Papillary Carcinoma

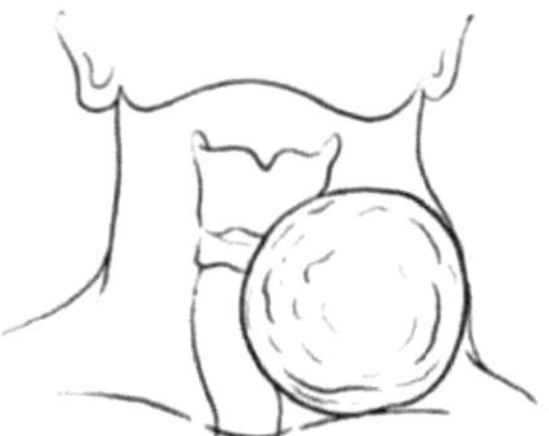

Fig. 49

T. N., a 28-year-old man was admitted to the hospital in January, 1971, with a mass in the anterior part of the neck of four years' duration.

Examination revealed a large, round tumor in the left lobe of the thyroid.   The size of the tumor was 6.5×7.5 cm and uniformly firm, with a smooth to slightly nodular surface (Fig. 49).   It was freely movable.   No lymph nodes were palpated in the neck.   Ultrasonic scanning revealed the tumor to be diffusely solid, and roentgenograms of the neck showed numerous psammomatous calcifications (Fig. 50).   Thus, an adenoma had been considered on the physical and ultrasonic examinations, but the roentgenographic finding strongly suggested the possibility of cancer.

At the time of operation, the left lobe of the thyroid contained a well encapsulated large tumor and there were no lymph node metastasis.   Hemithyroidectomy including a resection of the isthmus was performed.   (Figs. 51, 52).   Histologically the tumor was a papillary carcinoma of the thyroid with slight capsular invasion (Fig. 53).   The postoperative course was uneventful.

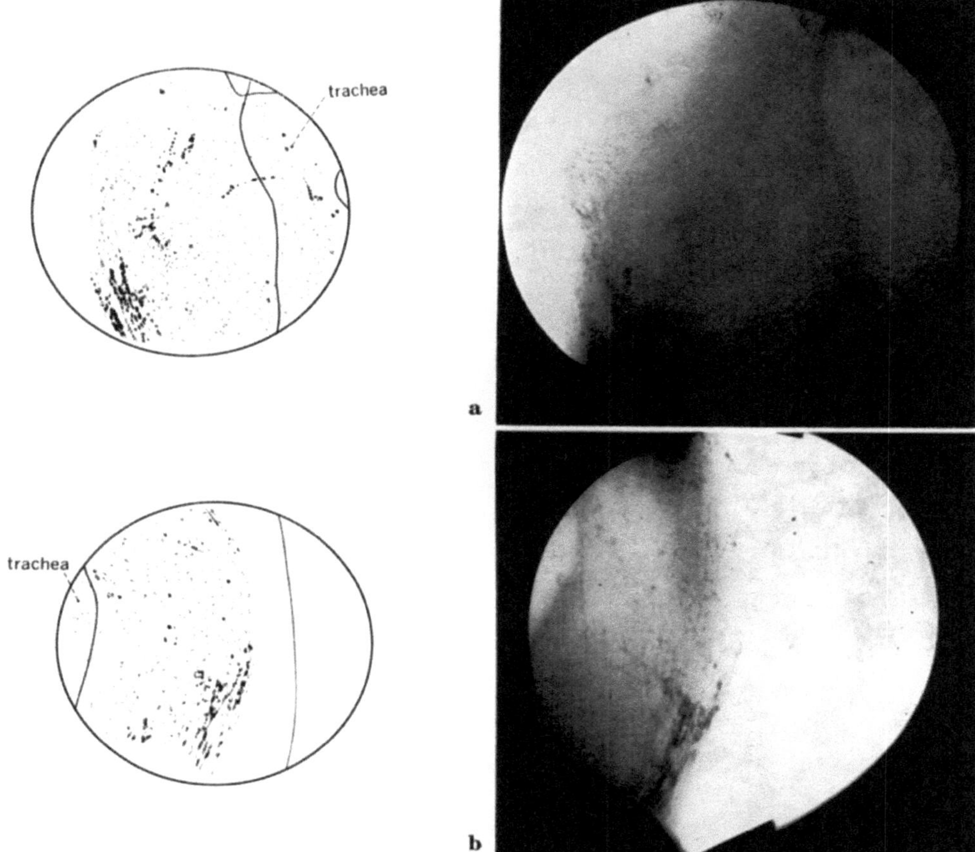

Fig. 50　Spot-tangential views of the neck.　Note typical psammomatous shadows.

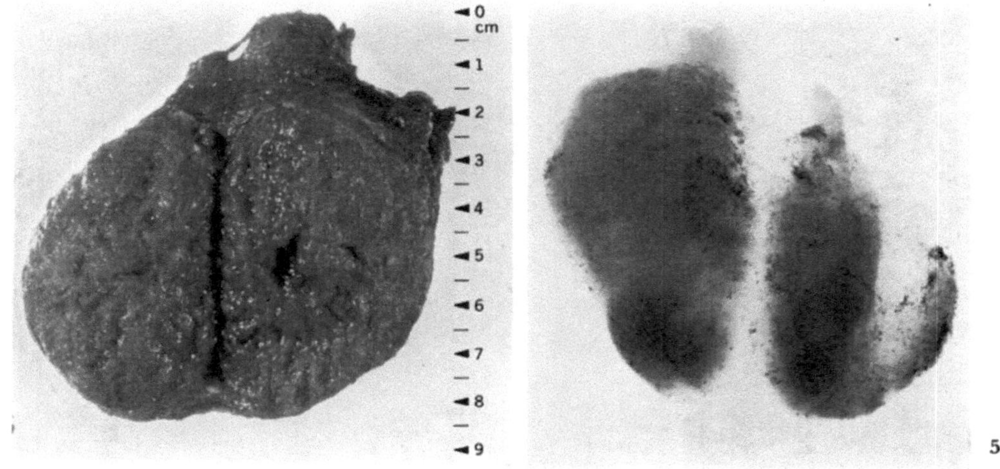

Fig. 51　Cut surface of the thyroid.　Macroscopically the tumor is well encapsulated.
Fig. 52　Roentgenogram of the surgical specimen, showing psammomatous pattern of calcification.

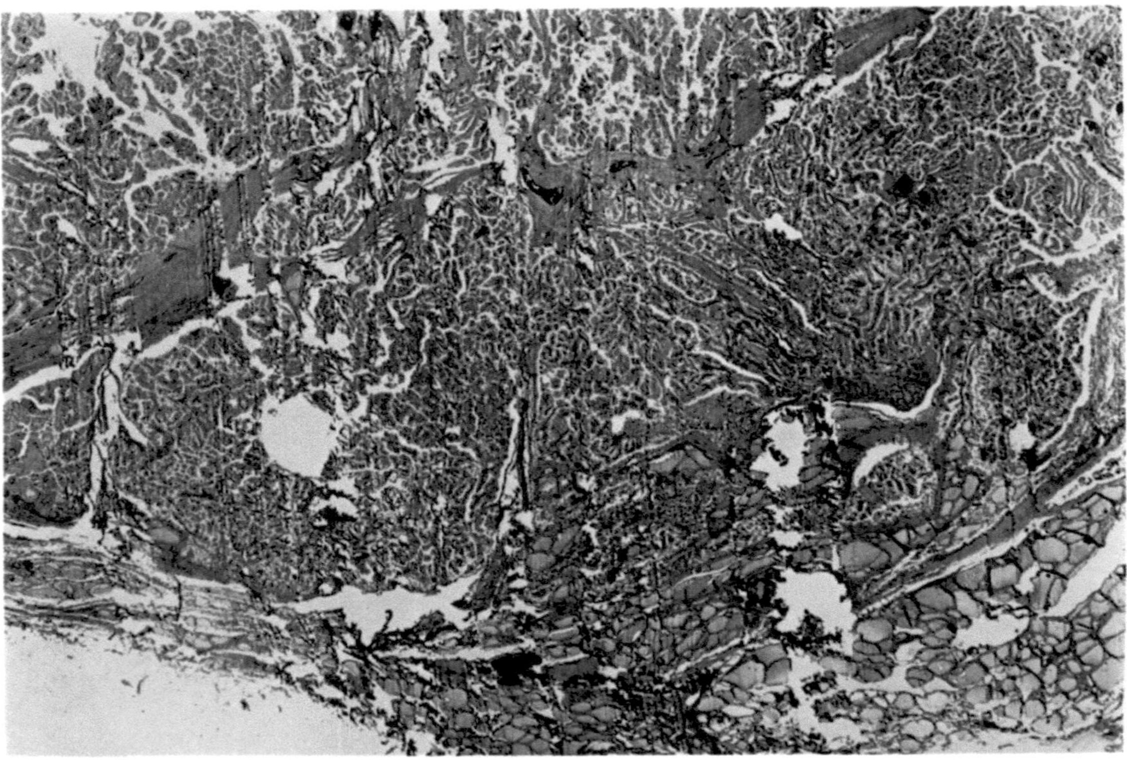

Fig. 53 Photomicrograph of specimen, showing a papillary carcinoma with slight capsular invasion. Aggregates of psammoma bodies are seen. The histologic section was damaged in cutting through the calcified area. (H & E, × 10).

Case 4. A Round Tumor Simulating an Adenoma: Papillary Carcinoma

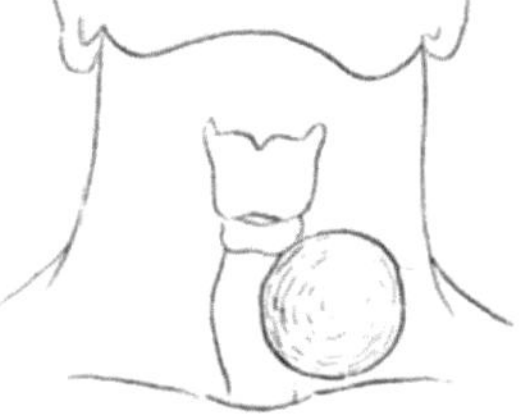

Fig. 54

M. S., a 29-year-old man first noticed a mass in the neck two years ago, which recently
increased in size despite medical treatment with desiccated thyroid. When he was referred to our institution for the evaluation of the nodule in June, 1971, there was a round,
smooth, easily movable, firm nodule 4 cm in diameter in the left lobe of the thyroid (Fig.
54). Ultrasonic scanning showed the solid nature of the tumor, and soft tissue roentgenograms of the neck revealed numerous psammomatous shadows (Figs. 55, 56). Thus, even
though the physical findings were those of a benign nodule, the roentgenographic finding
strongly indicated papillary carcinoma of the thyroid.

At the time of operation, the tumor was well encapsulated and a left lobectomy was
easily performed. On the cut surface of the removed specimen, it appeared grossly to be
a colloid adenoma (Fig. 57). The permanent paraffin sections revealed, however, papillary carcinoma with a mixed follicular and papillary pattern (Fig. 59). Capsular invasion
was minimal and the lymph nodes removed from the paratracheal area were negative for
malignancy.

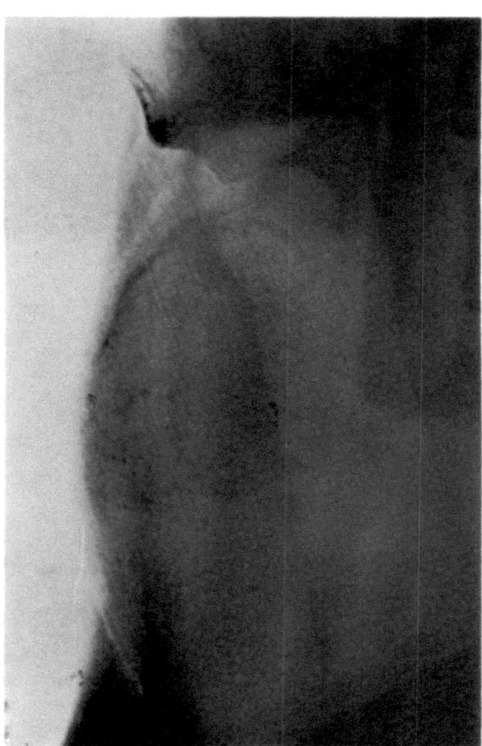

Fig. 55 Lateral view of soft tissue roentgenogram showing numerous calcium deposits in
a psammomatous pattern.

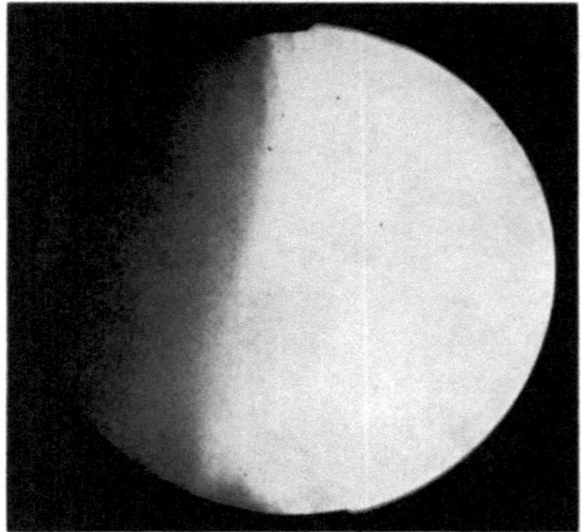
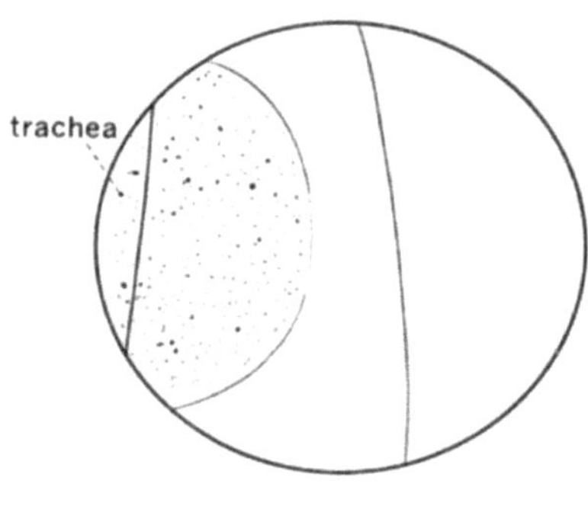

Fig. 56 Spot-tangential view demonstrating the psammomatous calcification more clearly.

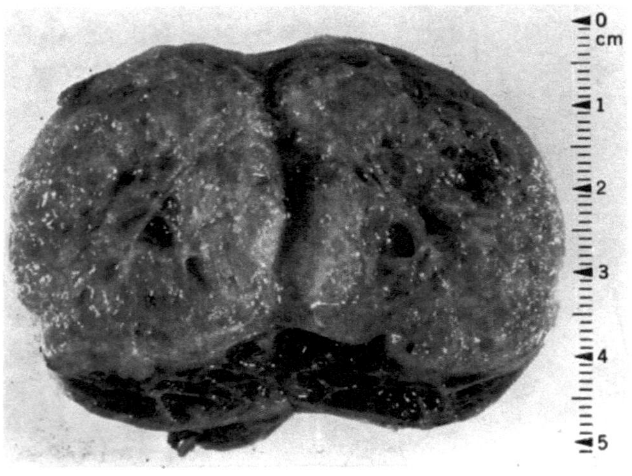

Fig. 57 Cut surface of the left lobe. The macroscopic appearance of the tumor is more like a colloid adenoma of the thyroid.

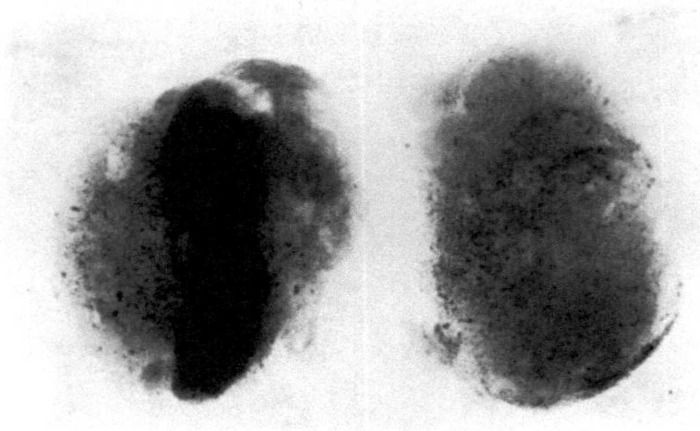

Fig. 58 Roentgenogram of specimen. Note typical psammomatous pattern of calcification.

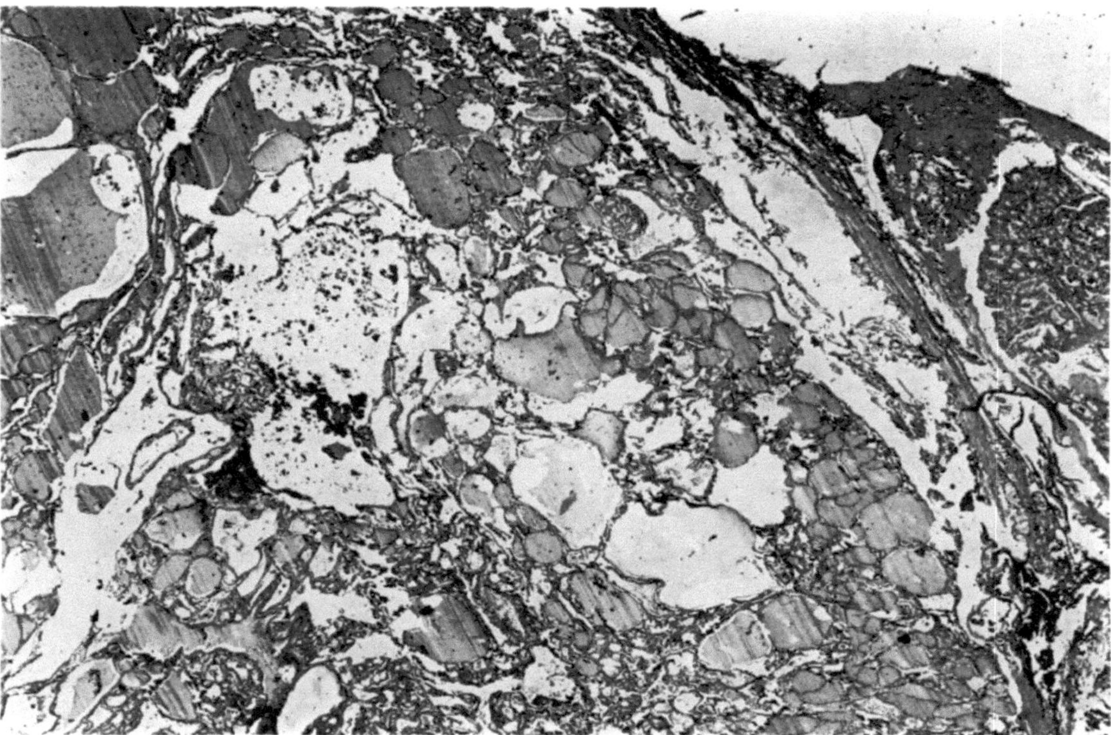

Fig. 59 Photomicrograph of specimen showing the papillary carcinoma with mixed macrofollicular and papillary pattern. Dust-like particles in the left upper portion are psammoma bodies. (H & E, ×10)

Case 5. A Small Round Tumor with a Rather Benign
Appearance: Papillary Carcinoma

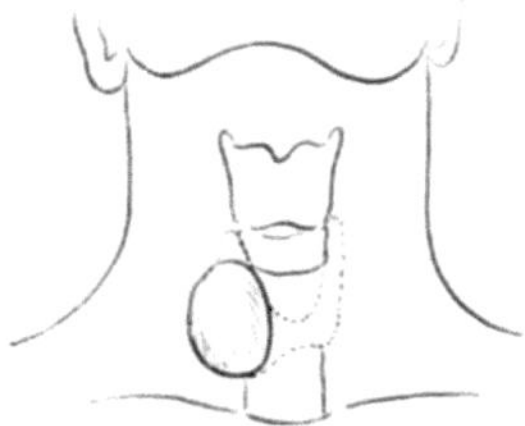

Fig. 60

K. T., a 23-year-old woman visited the hopital in August, 1970, with the complaint of a
mass in her anterior neck, which was noticed 5 years previously.

Examination revealed a firm, nodular mass in the right lobe of the thyroid. The mass
was 2×1.5 cm in size, oval with a smooth surface, and movable (Fig. 60). One surgeon
thought it to be an adenoma. However, one of the authors (Y. F.) thought that the
possibility of cancer could not be excluded, because the tumor was not readily movable
and the spot-tangential soft tissue roentgenogram of the neck disclosed the presence
of psammomatous calcification (Fig. 62).

At operation, the tumor proved to be a papillary carcinoma 1.5×1.8 cm in size,
the lesion being confined within the capsule of the thyroid gland (Fig. 63). The right
lobe and parathyroidal lymph nodes were removed. The postoperative course was uneventful. The pateint has been doing well with desiccated thyroid, 100 mg daily.

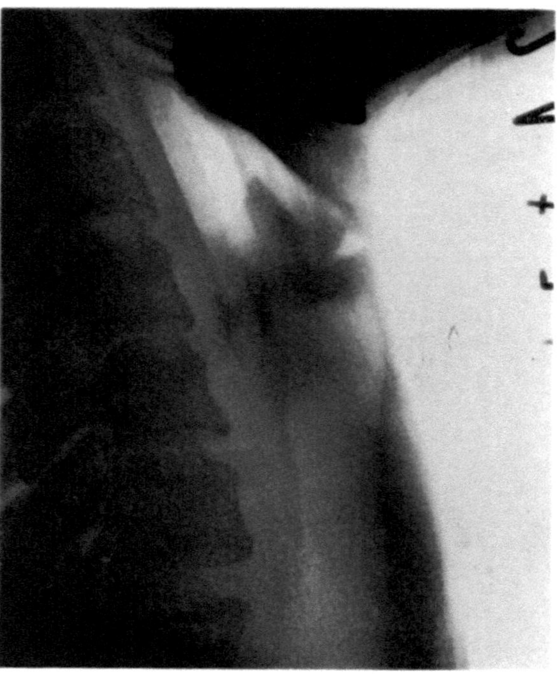

Fig. 61 Lateral soft tissue roentgenogram of
the neck. No calcifications are visible on this
film.

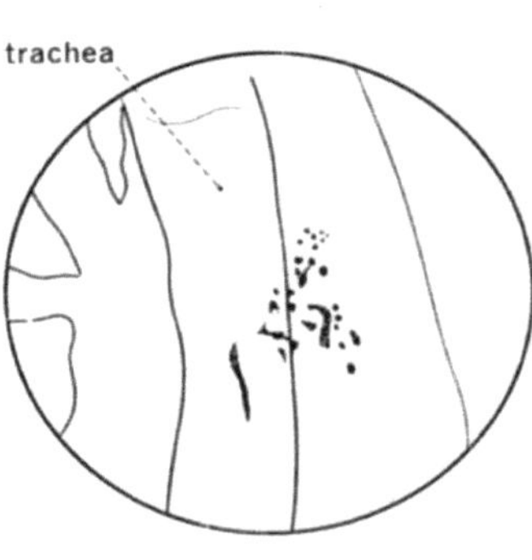

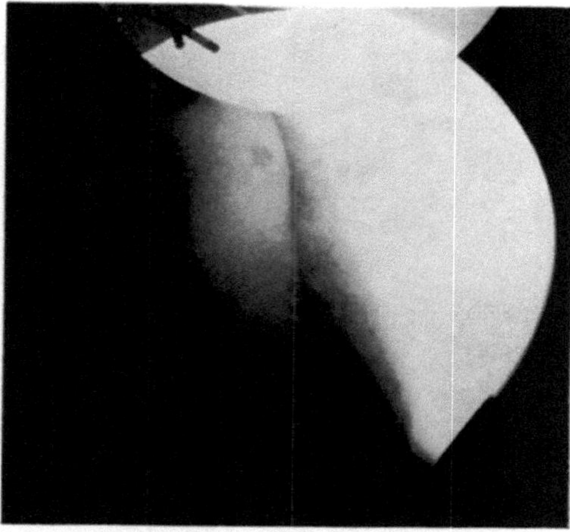

Fig. 62   Spot-tangential view demonstrating calcific shadows arranged in a pattern of thin strands and fine grains.

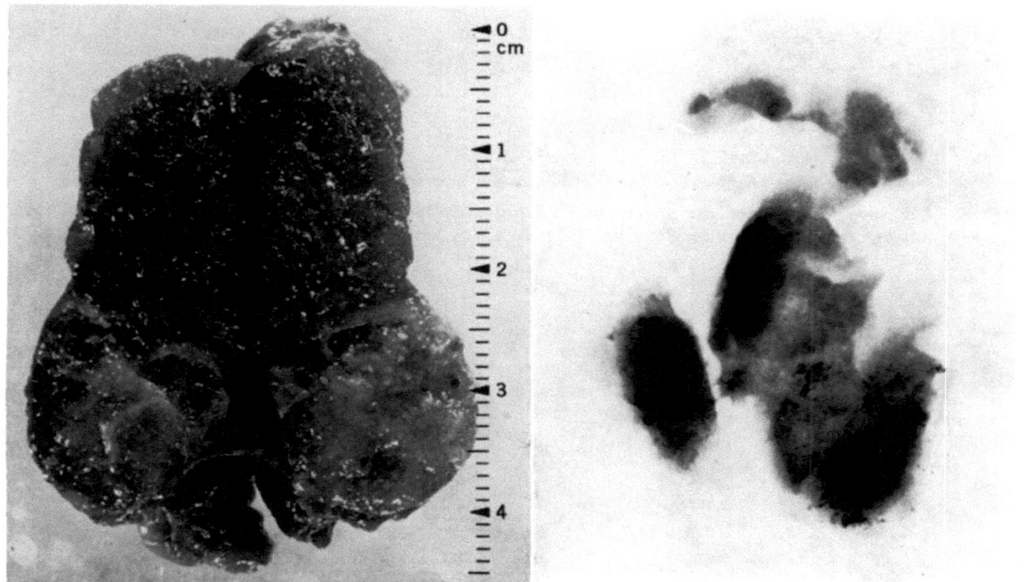

Fig. 63   Cut surface of the right thyroid lobe. The cancer is ocated in the lower portion of the lobe.
Fig. 64   Roentgenogram of the removed thyroid, showing psammomatous calcifications.

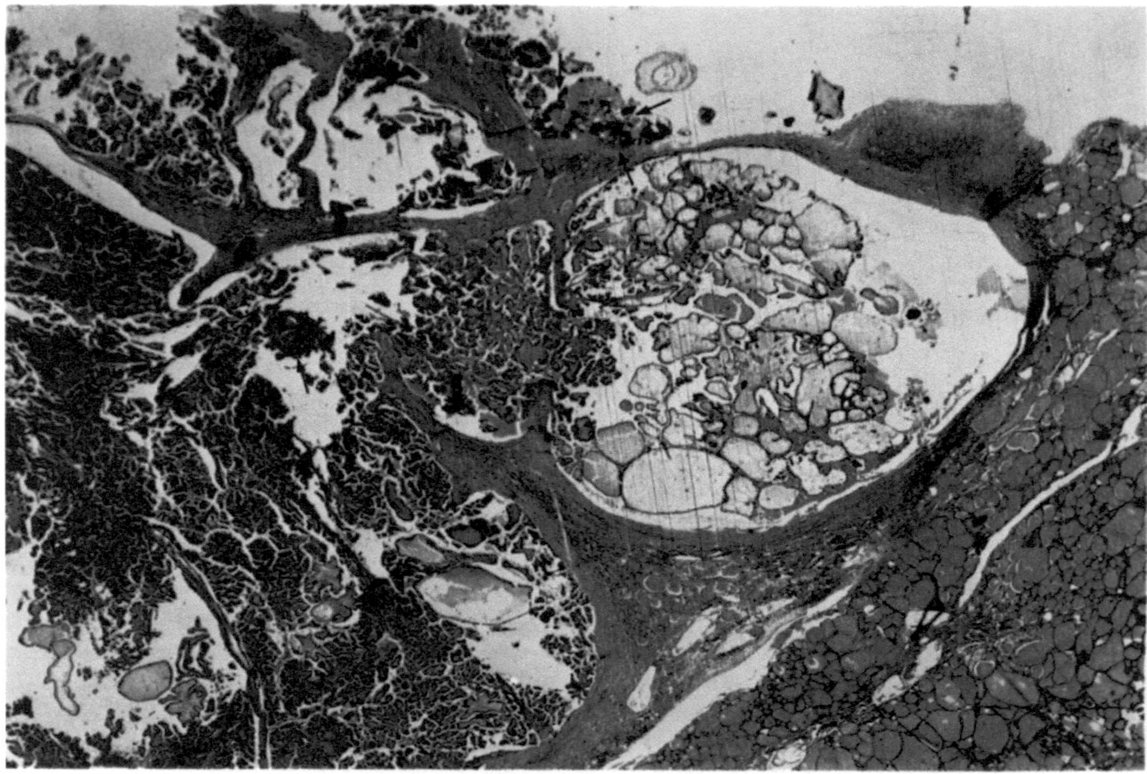

Fig. 65 Photomicrograph of the specimen showing papillary carcinoma of the thyroid containing aggregates of psammoma bodies. (H & E, ×10)

C. Miscellaneous Cases

Case 6. A Small Papillary Carcinoma with Jugular Lymph
Node Metastasis (Classified in Group III in Table
13)

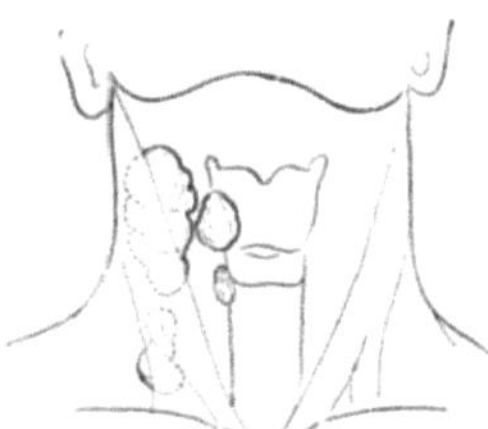

Fig. 66

N. O., a 26-year-old woman visited the hospital in April, 1971, complaining of a cold and slightly tender submaxillary lymph nodes.

Examination revealed multiple masses in the anterior and right lateral part of the neck. One of them was extremely hard, of small finger tip size and fixed to the thyroid cartilage. The others were apparently the enlarged lymph nodes of the deep jugular chain on the right side, which were adherent with each other, forming conglomerates. Careful palpation revealed a small tumor at the upper pole of the right lobe of the thyroid, which was hard and fixed to the trachea (Fig. 66).

The initial impression was the papillary carcinoma of the thyroid, but the possibility of tuberculosis of the cervical lymph nodes was also considered. The ESR was 8 mm per hour and chest x-ray examination disclosed no abnormal findings. Thyroid scintigram did not show any cold nodule (Fig. 67). [131]I thyroidal uptake at 24 hours was 19.8% and T_3 RSU was 31.4%. Soft tissue roentgenograms of the neck revealed distinct psammomatous calcification (Figs. 68, 70).

At operation, the 1×1.4 cm primary cancer was found in the right lobe, and the masses palpated preoperatively proved to be lymph nodes involved by metastases along the superior thyroidal artery and the internal jugular vein on the right side. All the lesions were removed by a subtotal thyroidectomy and modified radical neck dissection. Recovery following the operation was uneventful, except for a transient paralysis of the right vocal cord.

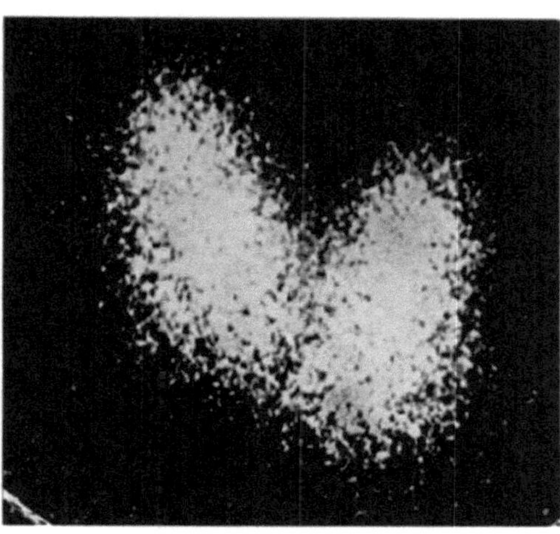

Fig. 67 Thyroid scintigram showing a diffuse uptake of radioiodine with no cold nodule demonstrated.

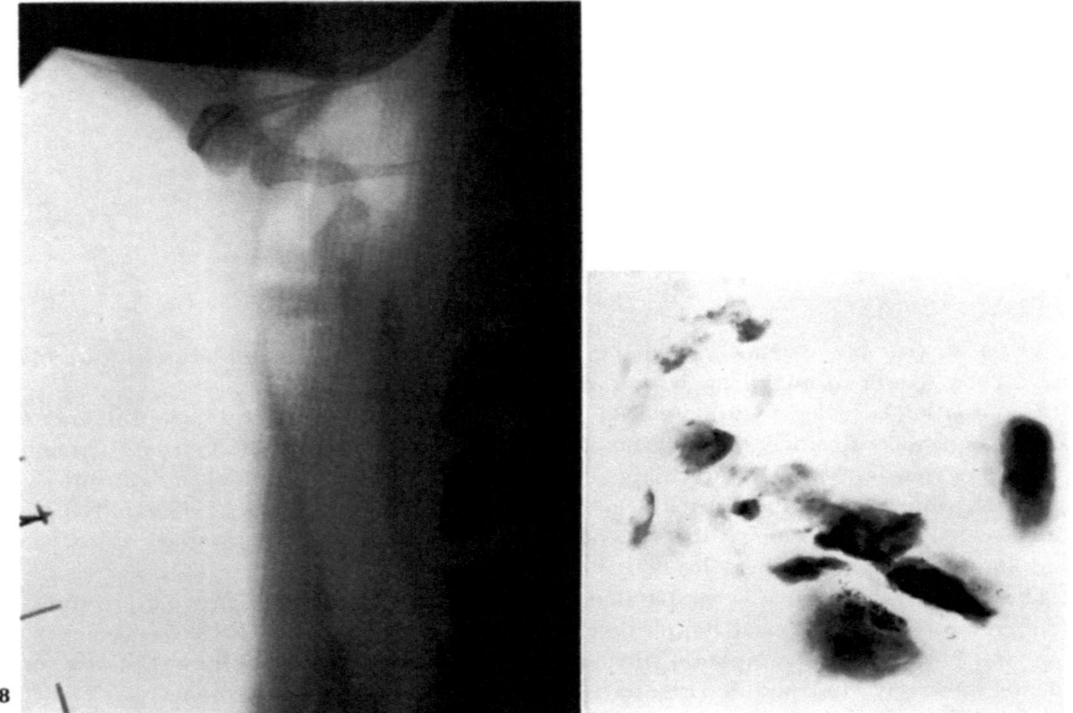

Fig. 68 Lateral soft tissue roentgenogram demonstrating a psammomatous pattern of calcification in the thyroid.

Fig. 69 Roentgenogram of the removed thyroid. Psammomatous calcification.

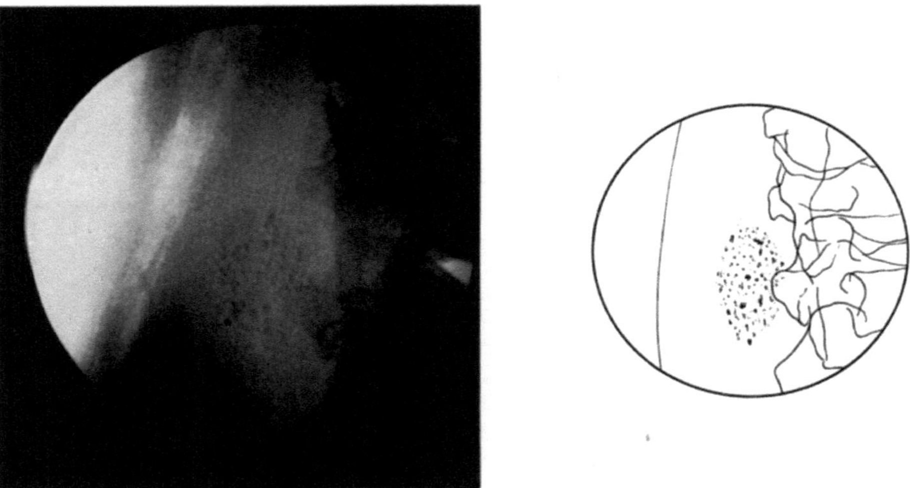

Fig. 70 Spot-tangential view showing more clearly defined psammomatous calcification.

Case 7. Papillary Carcinoma of the Thyroid Detected by Lymph Node Involvement (Classified in Group III in Table 13)

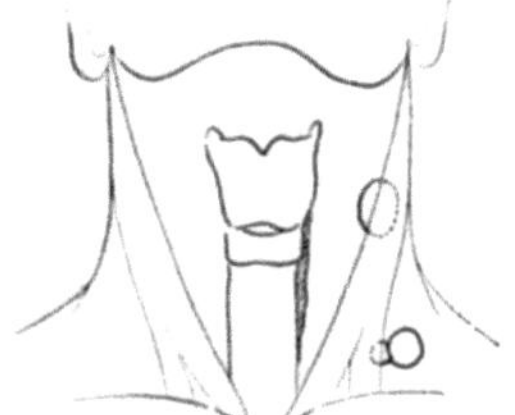

Fig. 71

I.M., a 44-year-old woman visited the hospital in July, 1969, with a complaint of lymph node swelling in the left cervical region of one month duration.   The patient had a history of previous operation for the enlarged lymph nodes in the neck probably due to tuberculous lymphadenitis 15 years previously.   At the outpatient clinic she was again diagnosed as having lymph node tuberculosis and was given chemotherapy until June, 1970, but the neck masses remained unchanged.   Chest x-ray and ESR at that time revealed no abnormal findings. An open biopsy was performed and histologic examination revealed lymph nodes involved with metastatic papillary carcinoma of the thyroid.

Careful, repeated physical examinations of the thyroid with knowledge of the pathological report disclosed only something like a fibrous thicknening a few milimeters in width along the left border of the trachea (Fig. 71).   Thyroid scintigram did not show a cold nodule.   A lateral view soft tissue roentgenogram of the neck did not show any calcified shadow (Fig. 72), but a spot-tangential view presented minimal, but definite psammomatous shadows (Fig. 73).

At operation, a carcinoma 1 cm in diameter was found in the upper pole of the left lobe.   Subtotal thyroidectomy and modified neck dissection were performed.   On the specimen roentgenogram, multiple but individually separated psammomatous calcifications were found within the tumor as well as in the neighboring thyroid parenchyma (Fig. 75).

Following the operation, she has been taking desiccated thyroid 100 mg daily and has remained well up to the present time.

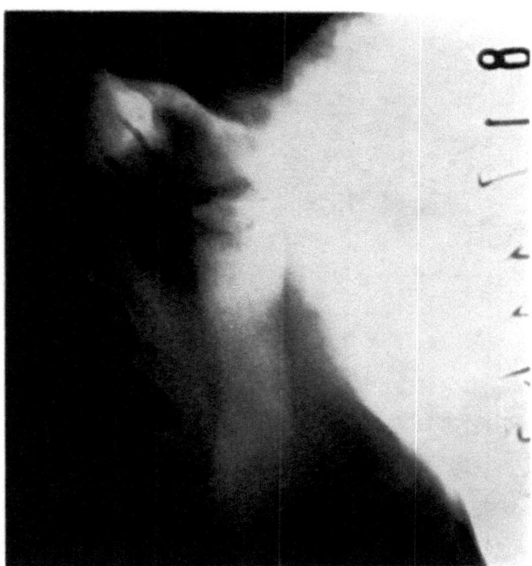

Fig. 72 Lateral soft tissue roentgenogram showing no calcific shadows in the thyroid region.

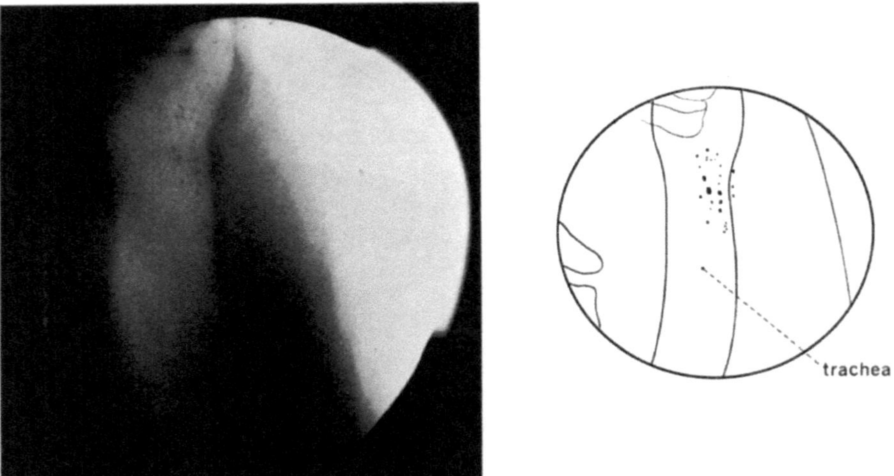

Fig. 73   Spot-tangential view demonstrating minimal but definite psammomatous calcifications.

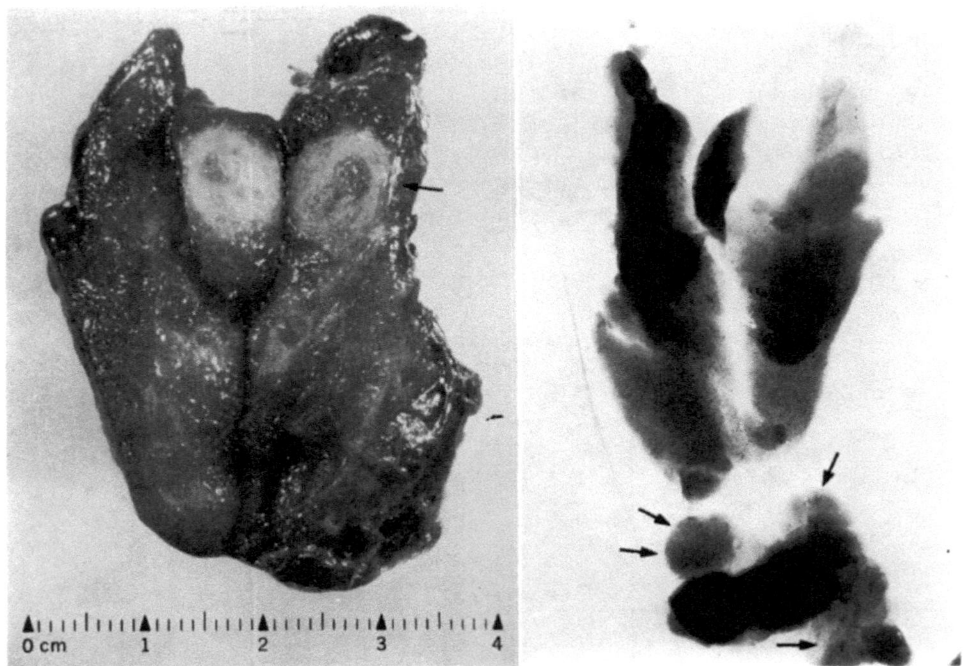

74   75

Fig. 74   Cut surface of the left lobe of the thyroid.   The primary cancer was 1 cm in diameter
and is seen in the upper portion of the lobe (arrow).

Fig. 75   Speciman roentgenogram showing a typical psammomatous pattern of calcification scattered
throughout the thyroid tissue.   Psammomatous calcific shadows (arrows) were also seen in the lymph
nodes involved by metastatic lesions.

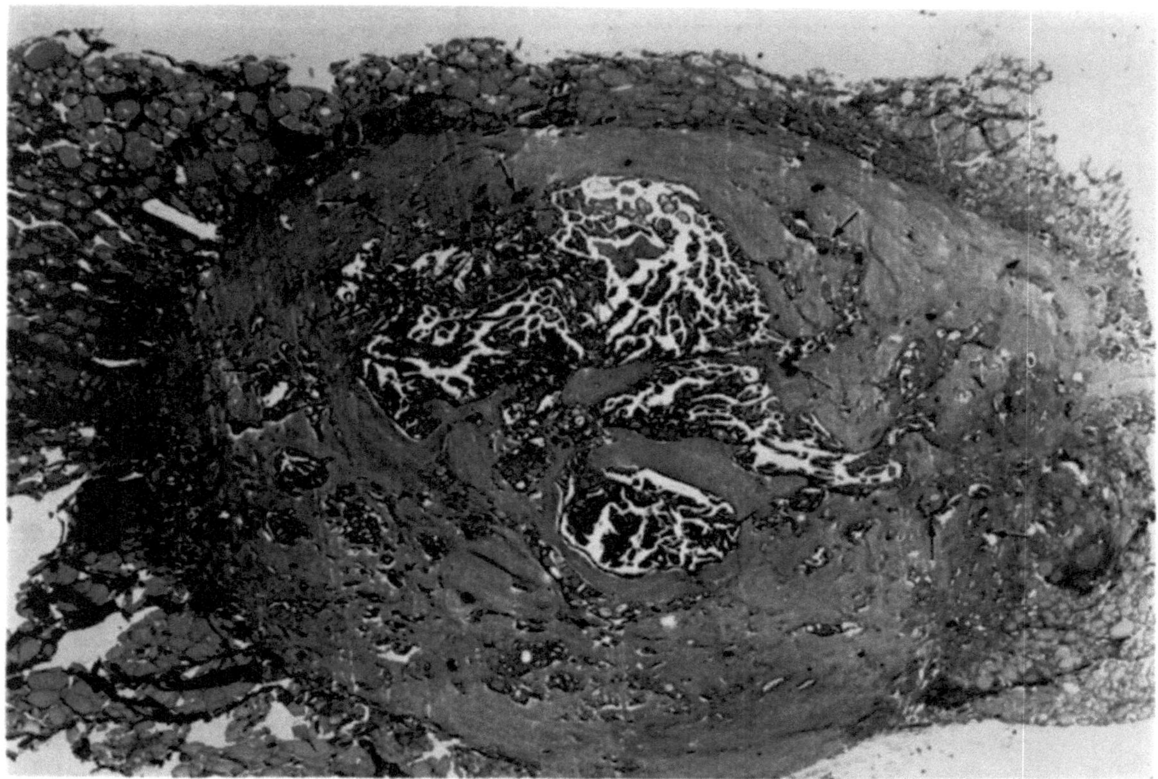

Fig. 76   Photomicrograph of specimen showing the primary lesion of papillary carcinoma. Psammoma bodies are seen as black grains.   (H & E, × 7)

Case 8. Papillary Carcinoma of the Thyroid Presenting as a Tender Nodule (Classified in Group II in Table 13)

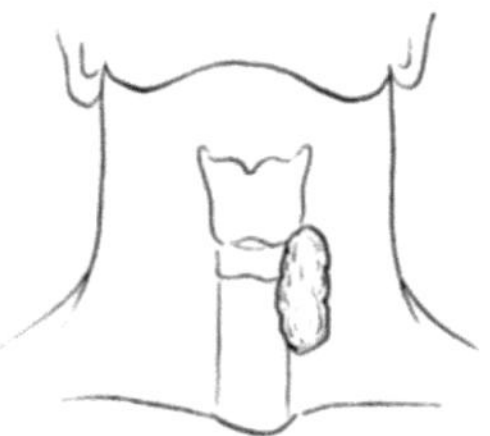

Fig. 77

O. K., a 43-year-old woman first noticed a tender mass in her anterior neck in late August, 1970.   On October 29, 1970, she was admitted to another hospital and was treated with prednisone and desiccated thyroid with the diagnosis of subacute thyroiditis.   On December 2, 1970, a thyroid scintigram was performed and a cold nodule with an irregular outline was found in the upper two thirds of the left lobe. ^{131}I thyroidal uptake at 24 hours was 11.3% and T_3 RSU was 28.0%. Because of these findings and the persistence of the nodule, the initial diagnosis of subacute thyroiditis was questioned and one of us (Y. F.) was asked to reevaluate the patient.

Physical examination revealed a 1.5×3 cm, firm, slightly movable nodule in the left lobe of the thyroid (Fig. 77).   On palpation, it was difficult to determine whether it was subacute thyroiditis or thyroid carcinoma.   However, ESR was normal and soft tissue roentgenogram of the neck showed both psammomatous and coarse clacifications (Figs. 78, 79), which was strongly indicative of thyroid carcinoma.

Subtotal thyroidectomy and a modified neck dissection were carried out on January 14, 1971.   The tumor proved to be the papillary carcinoma of the thyroid.

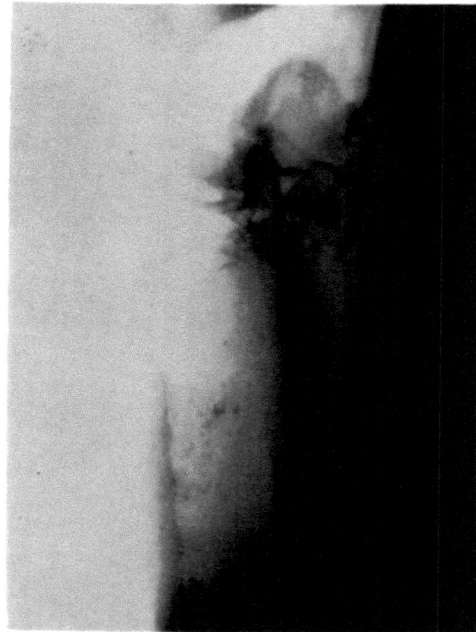

Fig. 78 Lateral soft tissue roentgenogram of the neck showing coarse calcific deposits combined with calcifications of a psammomatous pattern.

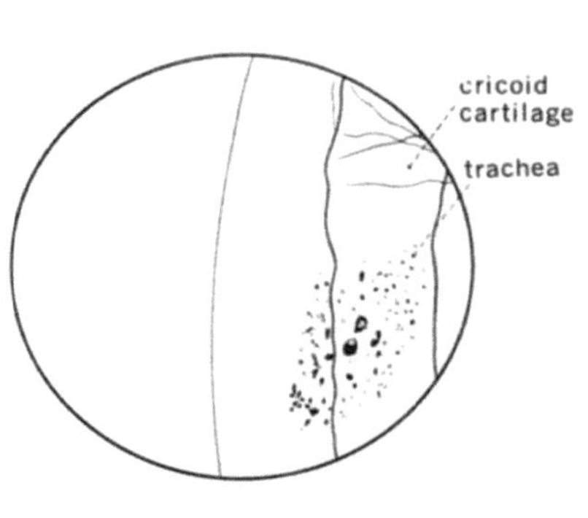

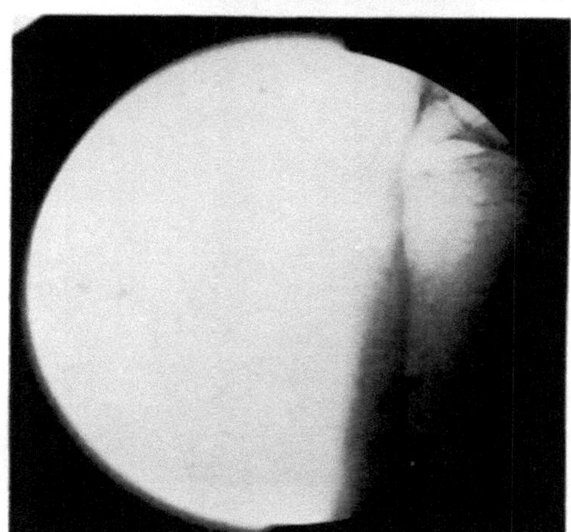

Fig. 79 Spot-tangential view showing more clearly defined thyroid calcification.

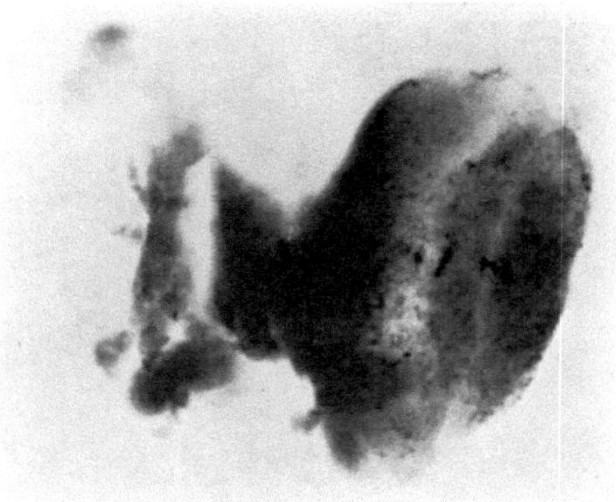

Fig. 80 Roentgenogram of removedthyroid. Coarse and psammomatous patterns of calcification are visible.

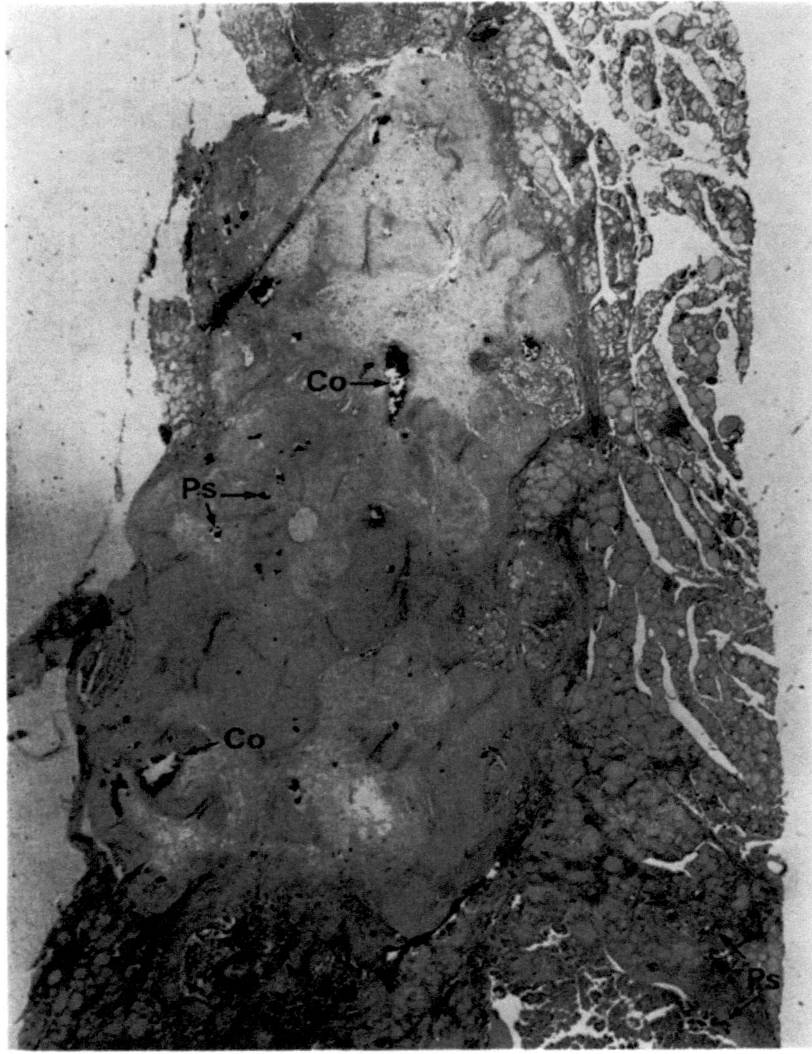

Fig. 81 Photomicrograph of specimen showing papillary carcinoma with areas of marked fibrosis. Coarse calcific deposits (Co) are in the area of fibrosis and the psammoma bodies (Ps) are in the papillary carcinoma tissue.   (H & E, ×10)

Case 9. Well-Encapsulated Follicular Carcinoma of the Thyroid (Classified in Group IV in Table 13)

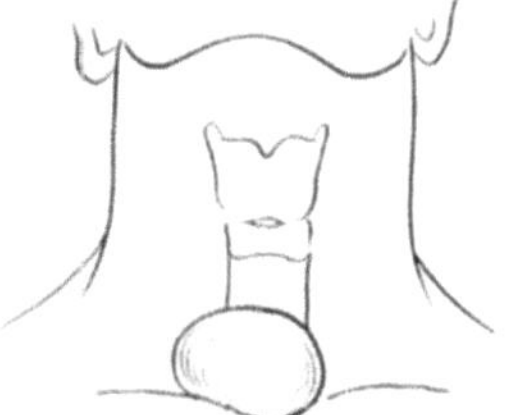

Fig. 82

A. I., a 56-year-old female was referred to us in September, 1970, from the Medical Department for evaluation of a thyroid nodule of two years' duration. Since she first noticed the nodule, it had continued to enlarge and recently she noticed a slight pressure sensation when swallowing.

Examination revealed an oval, firm, 3.5 × 5 cm mass in the anterior part of the neck just above the sternal notch (Fig. 82). Its surface was smooth, but it was not easily movable. Scintiscanning of the thyroid disclosed a smoothly outlined cold nodule in the lower portion of the right lobe, and ultrasonic scanning showed the tumor to be solid. Soft tissue roentgenograms of the neck showed both psammomatous calcifications and a long linear calcific deposit (Fig. 83). The latter finding was unusual for thyroid carcinoma.

At operation, the tumor was macroscopically well-encapsulated and was not adherent to the strap muscles or trachea. Subtotal thyroidectomy was easily carried out. Pathological examination revealed that the tumor was a follicular carcinoma with microscopic capsular invasion. The linear calcific deposit was found at the tumor capsule and psammomatous calcifications were due to the presence of both psammoma bodies and minute calcific deposits within the tumor stroma.

The patient has done well following surgery.

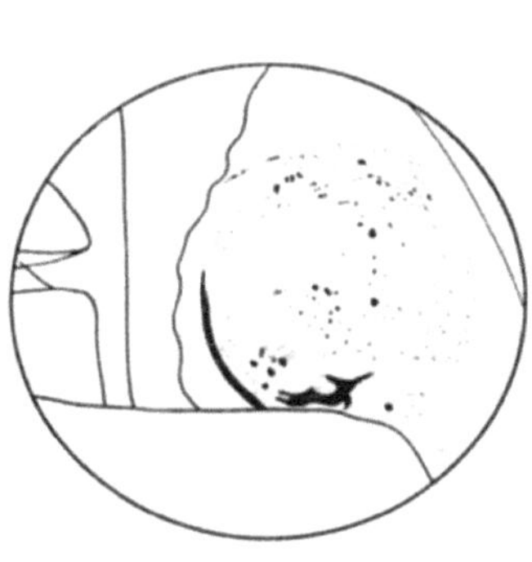

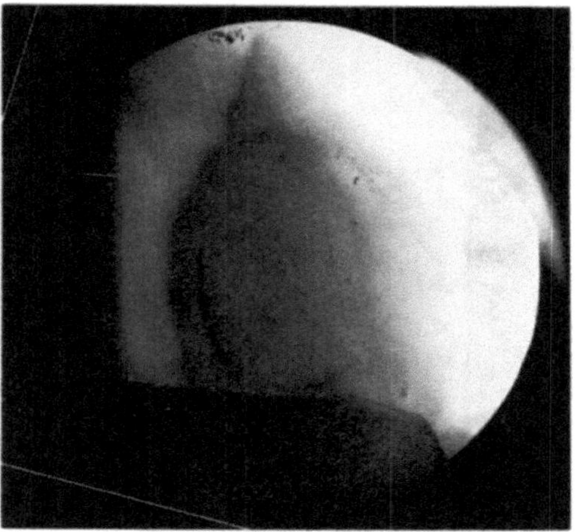

Fig. 83 Spot-tangential view of the neck, showing both curvilinear and psammomatous patterns of calcification.

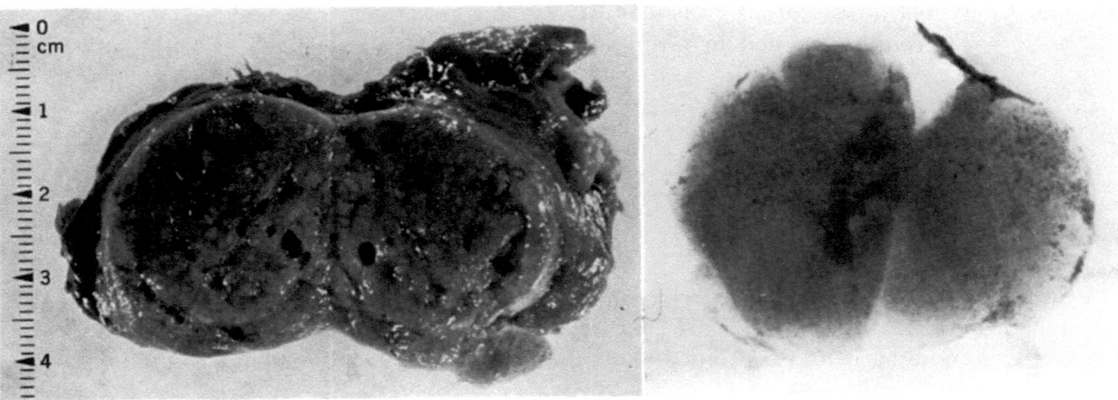

Fig. 84　　　　　　　　　　　　　　　　　　　Fig. 85

Fig. 84 Cut surface of the thyroid. The tumor is well encapsulated and macroscopically looks like a benign adenoma.

Fig. 85 Roentgenogram of the removed specimen. A typical psammomatous pattern of calcification is seen within the tumor parenchyma and the curvilinear calcific deposit is along the tumor capsule.

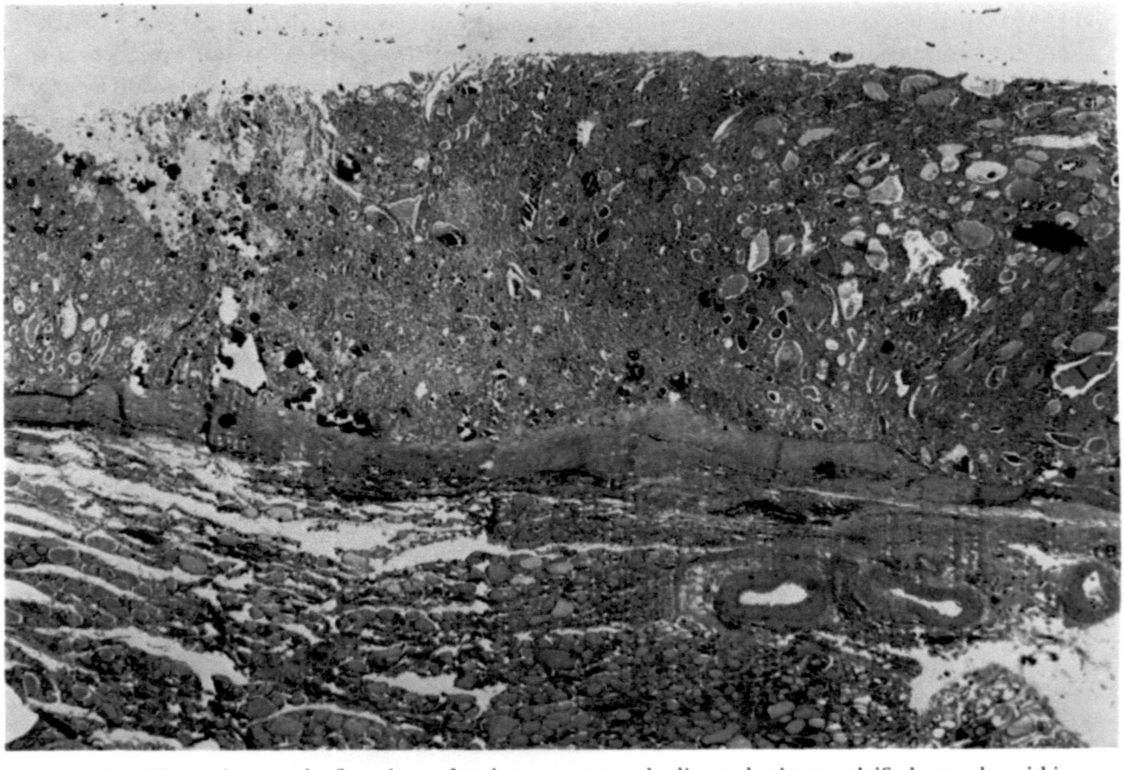

Fig. 86 Photomicrograph of specimen showing psammoma bodies and minute calcified granules within the tumor stroma. On this section, capsular invasion is not observed, but was apparent in other sections. (H & E, ×10)

II. CARCINOMA OF THE THYROID PRESENTING COARSE CALCIFICATION ALONE ON THE NECK FILMS

Case 10. A Firm, Non-Movable Nodule: Papillary Carcinoma (Group in II Table 13)

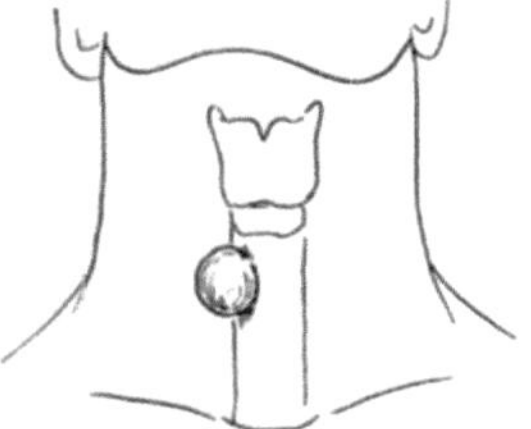

Fig. 87

S. Y., a 56-year-old woman noted a painless nodule in her anterior neck in early October, 1970. Shortly after that, when she visited the hospital a smooth, round, firm nodule approximately 1.5 cm in diameter was found in the right lobe of the thyroid which was fixed to the trachea (Fig. 87). Laboratory studies revealed an ESR of 29 mm per hour, ^{131}I thyroidal uptake at 24 hours of 2.1% and T_3 RSU of 26.7%. On the thyroid scintigram an irregular cold nodule was found in the right lobe. Ultrasonic scanning revealed a partly solid and partly cystic nodule. Soft tissue roentgenogram of the neck showed a coarse calcification (Fig. 88). From these results, a papillary carcinoma of the thyroid with cyst formation was suspected preoperatively and this impression was confirmed at the time of operation.

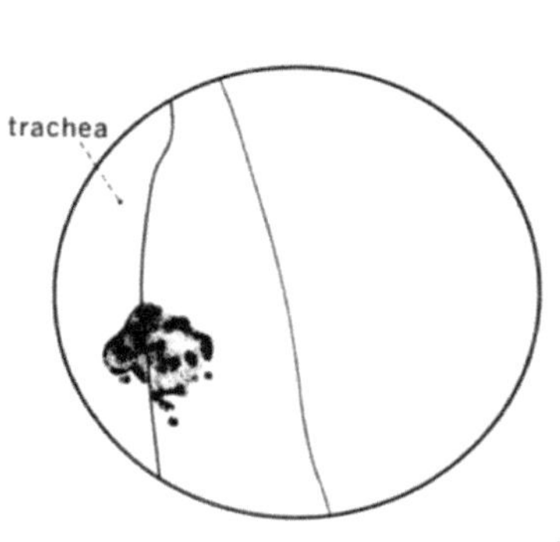

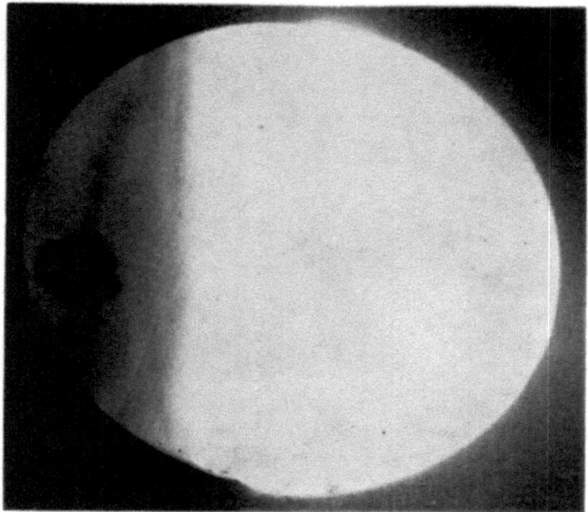

Fig. 88 Spot-tangential view demonstrating a dense calcium deposit.

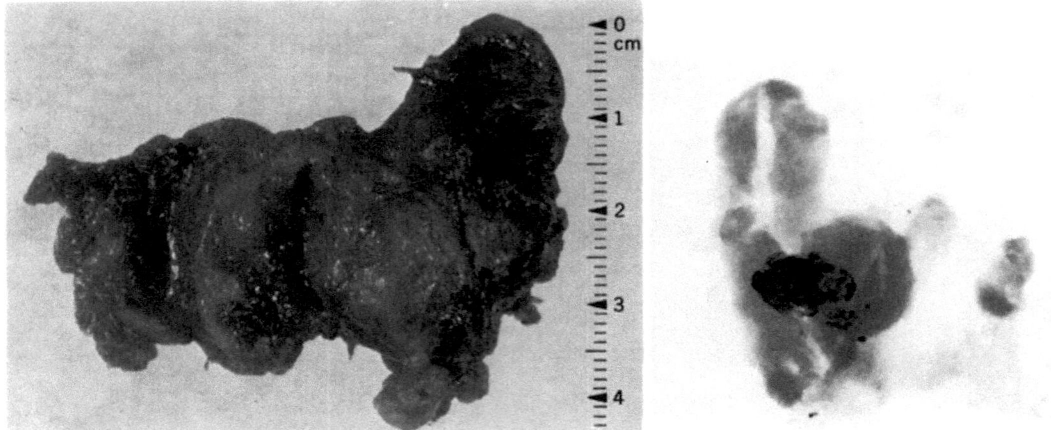

89   90

Fig. 89   Removed thyroid specimen, showing the cut surface of the tumor.
Fig. 90   Roentgenogram of the removed specimen.

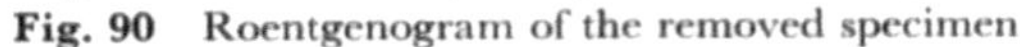

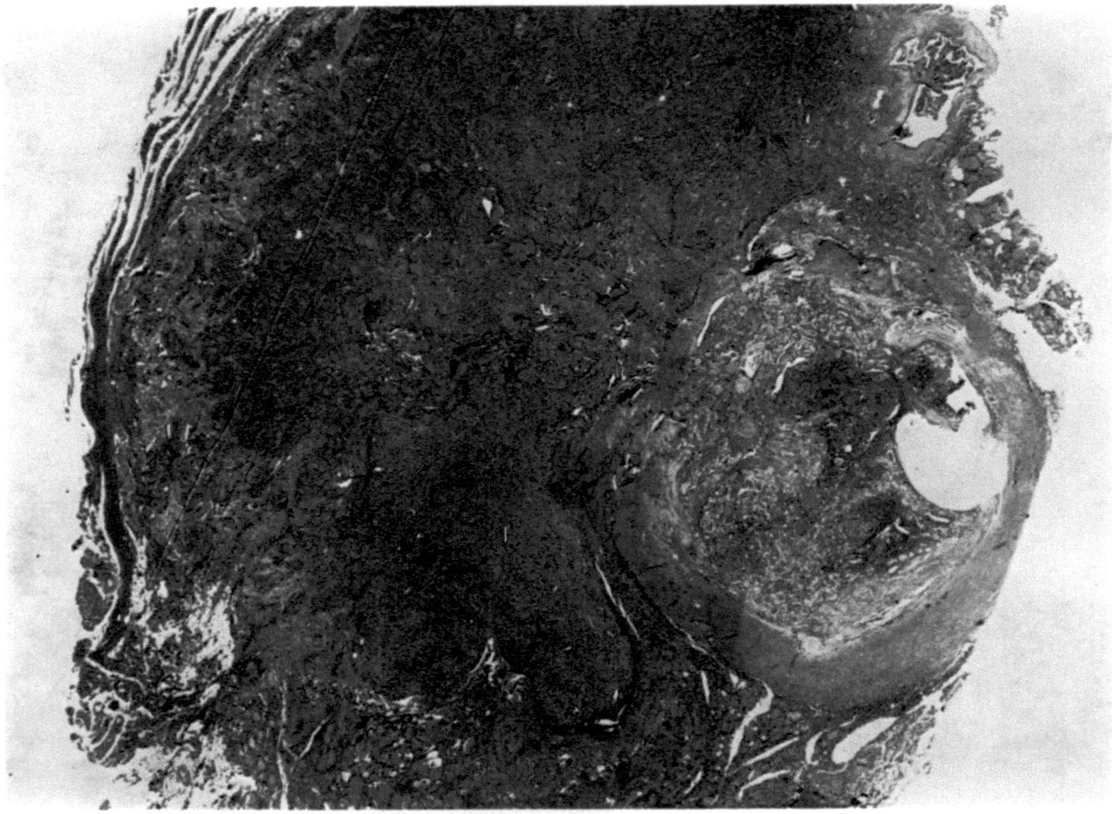

Fig. 91   Photomicrograph of specimen, showing papillary carcinoma of the thyroid with marked capsular invasion.   On this section, a small cystic cavity is visible within the encapsulated portion of cancer.   The massive deposit of calcium occurred in the fibrous capsule.   (H & E, × 7)

Case 11. Recurrent Hard Nodule with a Cystic Protrusion:
Papillary Carcinoma (Group II in Table 13)

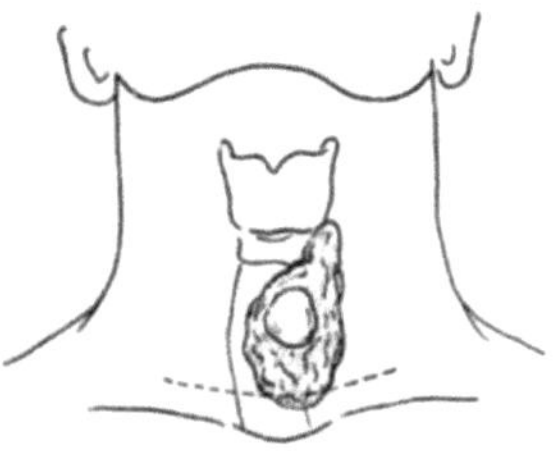

Fig. 92

Y. G., a 59-year-old woman visited the hospital in October, 1970, complaining of re-
currence of a tumor in her anterior neck of 10 months' duration. A thyroid operation
had been preformed by another surgeon 10 years previously, which was followed by
postoperative irradiation.

Examination revealed an iron-hard, fixed, irregular mass 4×4 cm in size in the
left lobe of the thyroid. A cystic nodule, about 1.5 cm in diameter, protruded anteriorly
from this hard mass, which was the major complaint of the patient (Fig. 92). No lymph
nodes were found in the neck. Laryngo-tracheoscopic examination revealed that the
movement of vocal cords was normal bilaterally and no tumor mass was found on the
tracheal mucosa. Thyroid function tests showed ^{131}I thyroidal uptake at 24 hours of 17.8
% and T_3 RSU of 29.7%. Roentgenograms of the neck showed massive deposits of calcium in the mass (Figs. 93, 94). All of these findings indicated that the tumor was most
likely a papillary carcinoma of low grade malignancy and should be resectable.

At the time of operation, it was found that the cancer had not invaded the trachea,
but only fibrous adhesions were present between the tumor and the trachea, so the radical
operation was successfully carried out. Subtotal thyroidectomy and a modified neck dissection on the left side were performed without complication.

The patient has been given suppressive doses of desiccated thyroid and has remained
well until the present time.

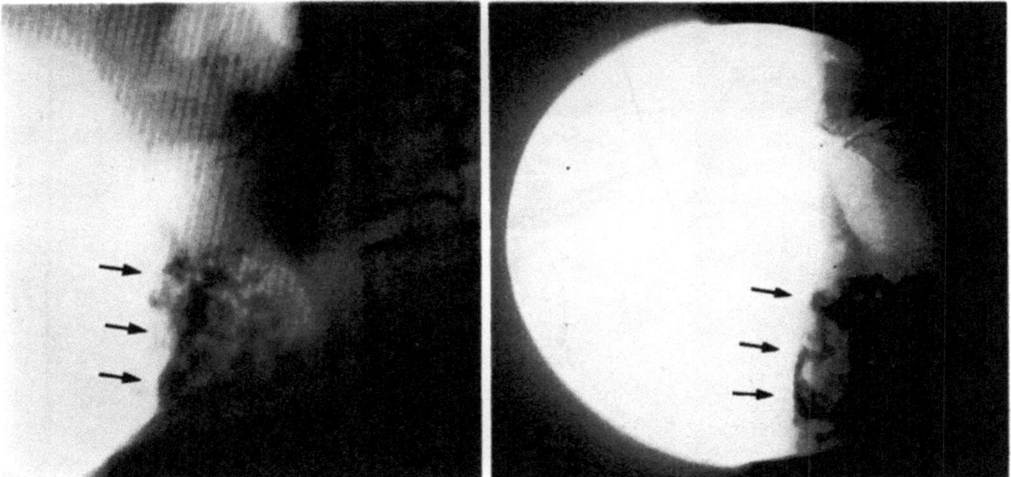

93   94

Fig. 93 Lateral standard roentgenogram of the neck. A massive amorphous deposit of calcium is
evident (arrows).

Fig. 94 Spot-tangential view. Calcific deposits (arrows) are much more clearly defined than on the
conventional roentgenogram.

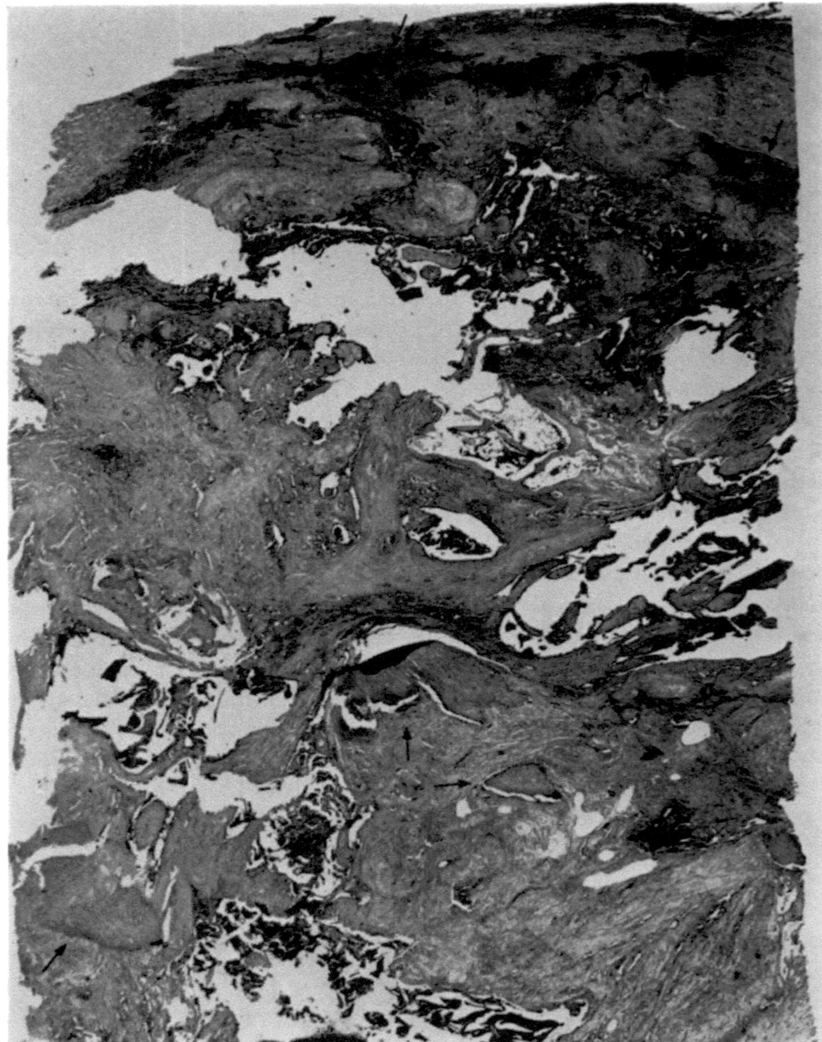

Fig. 95   Photomicrograph of the specimen showing papillary carcinoma of the thyroid with multiple areas of fibrosis, where calcium deposition occurred (arrows).   (H & E, $\times$ 20)

Case 12. A Hard, Irregular Mass: Papillary Carcinoma
(Group II in Table 13)

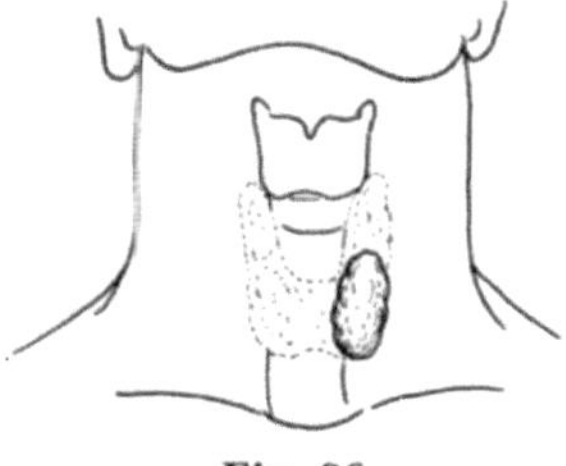

Fig. 96

A. P., a 42-year-old woman with the past history of three abdominal operations visited another hospital in May, 1970, complaining of dull pain in the right lower abdomen and a thyroid nodule was detected by a physician. Five months later she was referred to us for evaluation of the thyroid nodule.

Examination revealed a hard, irregular, slightly movable mass measuring 1.5×2 cm, located in the lower portion of the left lobe (Fig. 96). ^{131}I thyroidal uptake was 8.9 %, T_3 RSU was within normal limits, and a cold nodule was shown on the scintigram. Roentgenograms of the neck showed multiple coarse calcific deposits of irregular shape (Fig. 97). A carcinoma of the thyroid was suspected.

At the time of operation, there was a well-encapsulated, densely calcified, hard mass approximately 2 cm in diameter in the middle of the left lobe, which was macroscopically thought to be a benign nodule. In addition, a hard nodule less than 1 cm in diameter was found in the upper pole of the same lobe (Figs. 98, 99). A left lobectomy was performed. Pathologic examination revealed that the lower larger nodule to be an encapsulated papillary carcinoma (Fig. 100), and the upper smaller one to be a 0.8 cm, occult carcinoma (Fig. 101). When the roentgenograms of the neck was reviewed retrospectively, a coarse calcific deposit was detectable at the site corresponding to the occult carcinoma.

The patient has been under the treatment with suppressive doses of desiccated thyroid and has remained well.

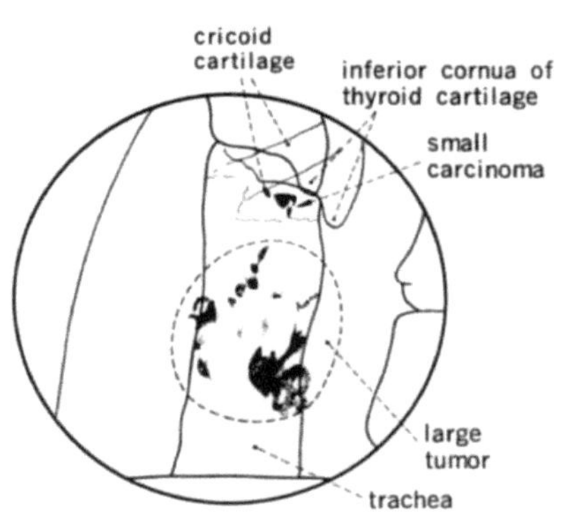

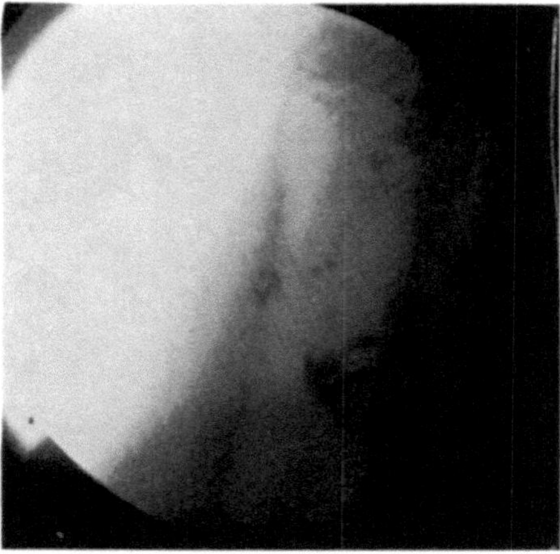

Fig. 97 Spot-tangential view of the neck. Coarse calcifications with a variety of configulations seen on this film are similar to the pattern usually observed in cases of adenomatous goiter, such as shown in Fig. 134, 138 and 141. However, the physical findings of the neck mass indicated a malignant lesion. Retrospective review of this film revealed that the uppermost carcification just inferior to the cricoid cartilage was actually in the isolated small cancer incidentally found at operation.

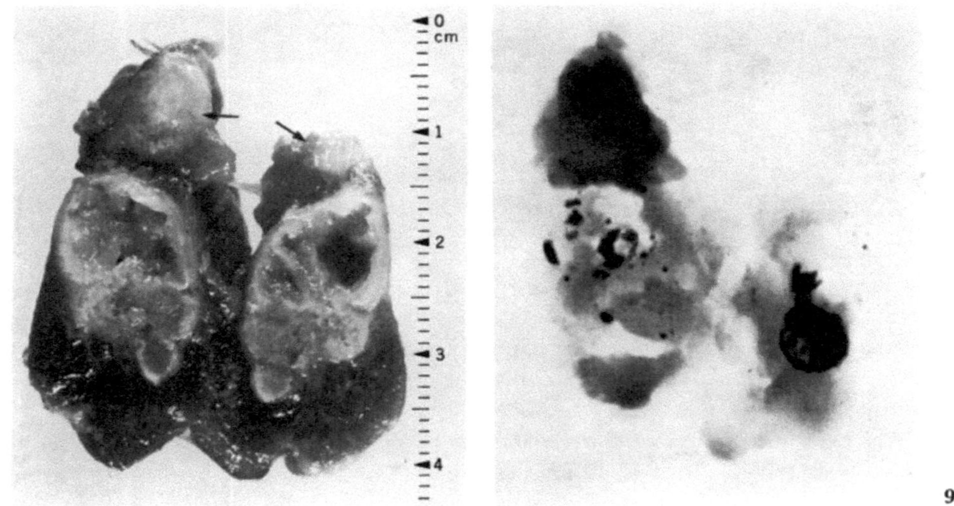

Fig. 98   Cut surface of the left lobe.   A sharply demarcated 2 cm nodule with a thick fibrous capsule is located in the middle of the lobe, and another small hard nodule is present in the upper pole (arrow).

Fig. 99   Roentgenogram of the removed specimen.   Coarse calcifications are seen in both nodules.

Fig. 100   Microscopic appearance of the lower, larger nodule; an encapsulated papillary carcinoma. Calcific deposits are seen in the fibrous capsule.   (H & E, × 15)

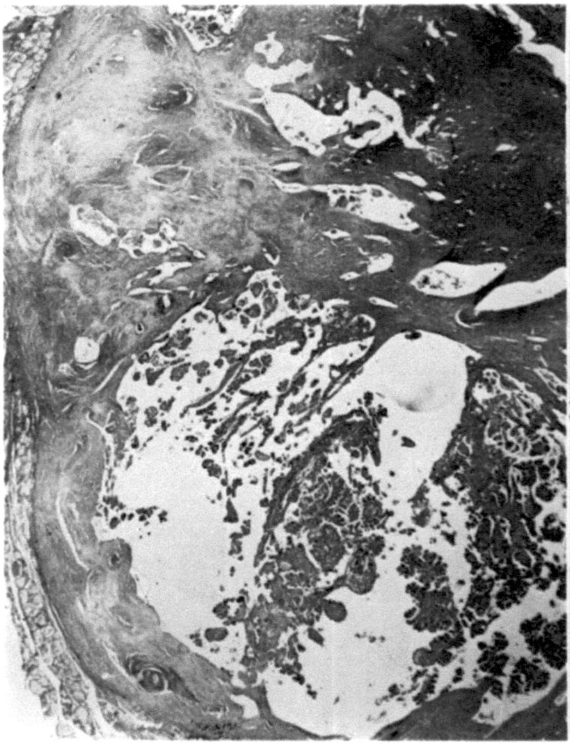

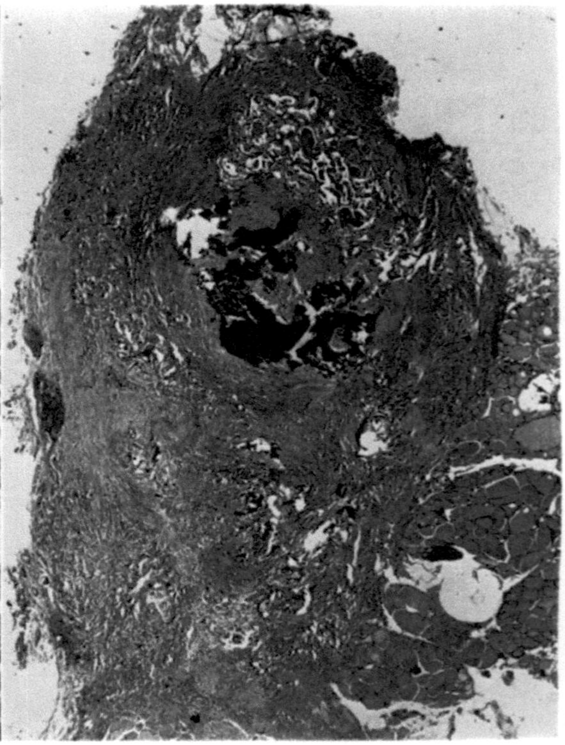

Fig. 101   Microscopic section of the upper, smaller nodule; papillary carcinoma with areas of calcified fibrosis.   (H & E, × 15)

Case 13. Follicular Carcinoma of the Thyroid with Metastases to Lymph Nodes and Lung of Long Dura-
tion (Group I in Table 13)

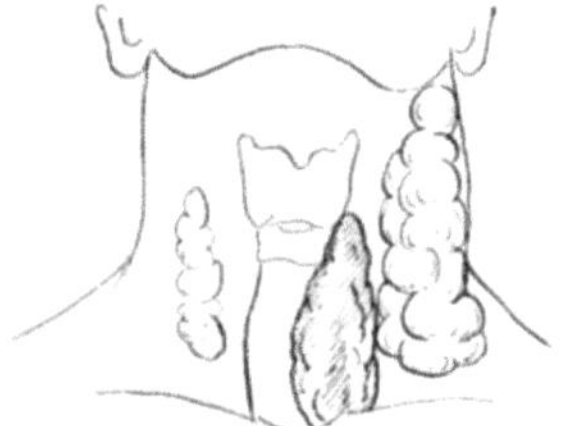

Fig. 102

M. T., a 68-year-old man came to the hospital in July, 1971, with the chief complaint of multiple neck masses of 40 years' duration and recent onset of neuralgic pain in the left lateral aspect of the neck. The masses had gradually increased in size for the first 15 years and then remained almost the same size. He was told that there were a great number of miliary deposits spread evenly throughout his lungs on a chest x-ray 15 years previously, but the nature of these lesions was not determined. Since that time periodic chest x-rays have shown no progression of the lesions.

Examination revealed multiple bilateral enlarged lymph nodes in the neck, more marked on the left. A hard 4 × 5.5 cm tumor was found in the left lobe of the thyroid, which was firmly fixed to the trachea (Fig. 102). Chest x-ray showed multiple, sharp-ly circumscribed, small nodules scattered widely throughout both lungs and a mass lesion in the right upper mediastinum (Figs. 103, 104). On the anteroposterior view of the neck, deviation of the trachea toward the right and widening of the right upper medi-astinum were evident (Fig. 105). Lateral and spot-tangential views of the neck revealed coarse calcifications in both the thyroid lesion and the involved lymph nodes (Figs. 106, 107, 108). Radioiodine scintiscanning of the neck and chest disclosed uptake of ^{131}I in the metastatic lesions of the bilateral jugular lymph nodes, right upper mediasti-num and both lungs (Figs. 109, 110).

The patient looked quite healthy and euthyroid. Laboratory studies were BMR of +4%, normal blood cell counts, alkaline phosphatase of 11.2 King Armstrong units and LDH of 308 units.

Subtotal thyroidectomy and removal of the affected lymph nodes through the original collar incision were carried out in January, 1972. Histologic sections revealed well differentiated carcinoma of follicular and papillary pattern. No areas of anaplastic car-cinoma were found. He has been treated with a replacement dosage of desiccated thyroid and has been doing well.

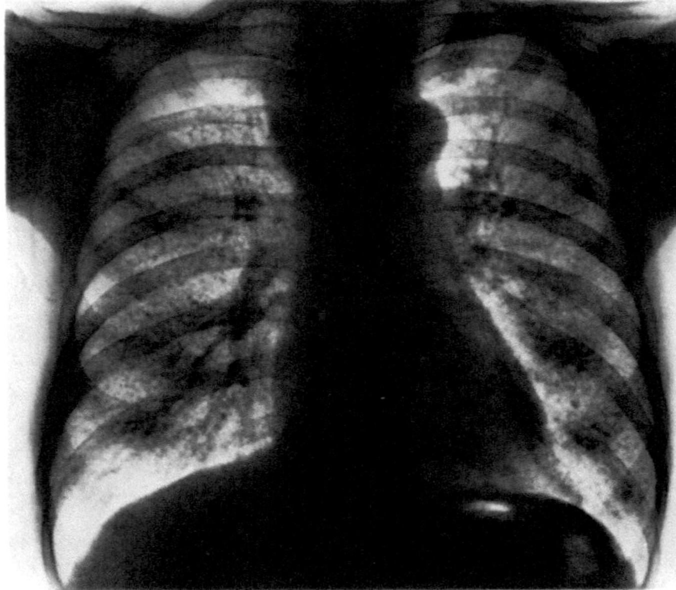

Fig. 103 Chest x-ray showing miliary deposits throughout the both lungs, deviation of the trachea toward the right, and widening of the right upper mediastinum.

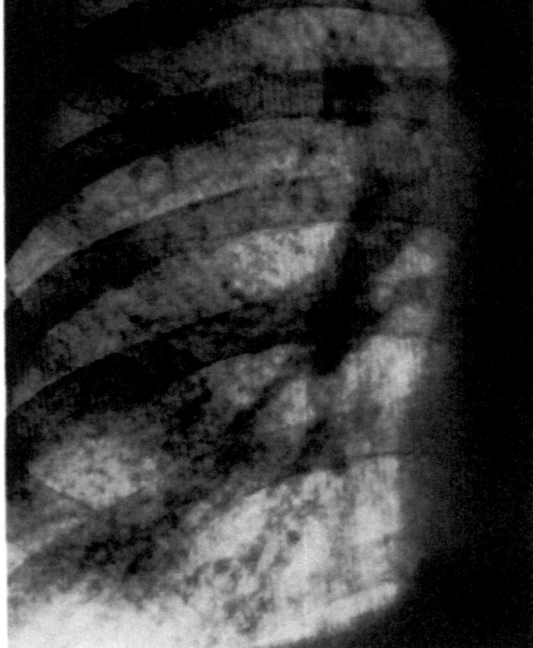

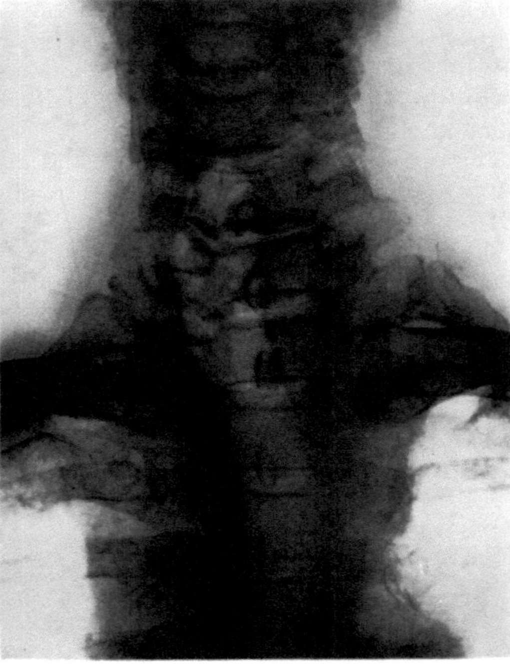

Fig. 104 Mid-portion of the right lung. Note the miliary deposits; one of the typical patterns of pulmonary metastasis from well-differentiated thy-

Fig. 105 Antero-posterior view of the neck. Deviation of the trachea toward the right is evident, but no narrowing of tracheal lumen is observed.

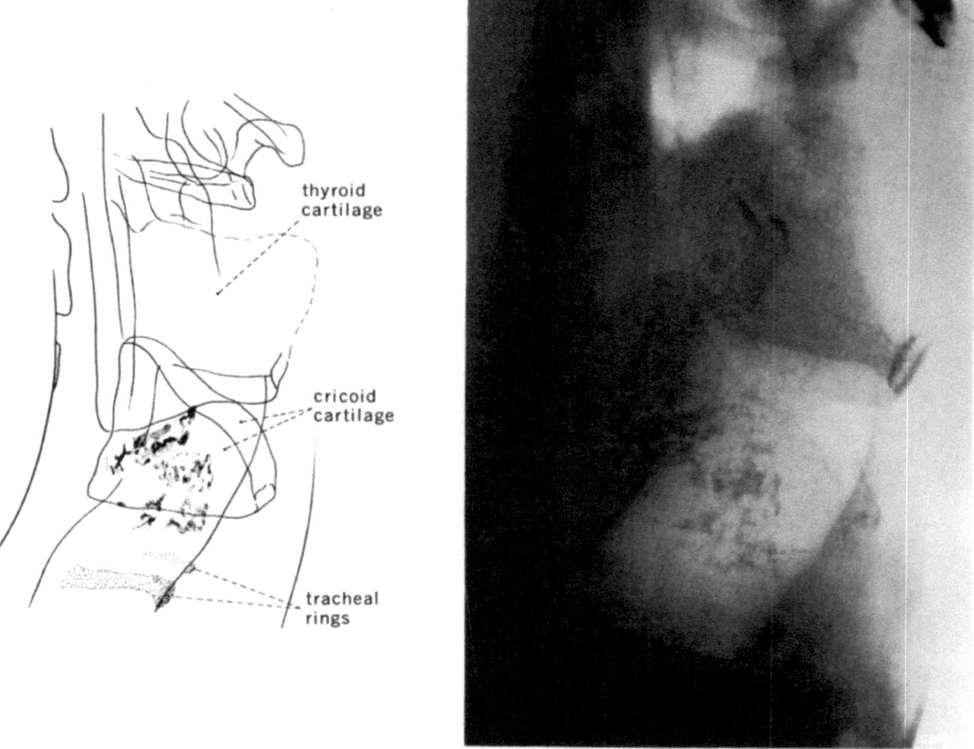

Fig. 106   Lateral soft tissue roentgenogram of the neck, showing amorphous calcific deposits.

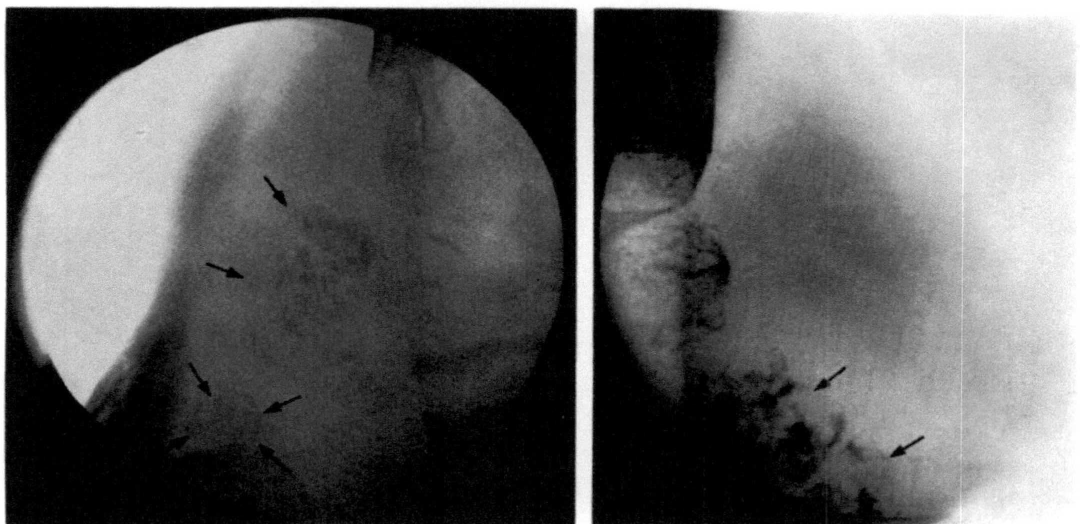

Fig. 107, 108   Spot-tangential views showing irregular coarse calcifications arranged in a punctate and amorphous pattern.

CASE REPORTS

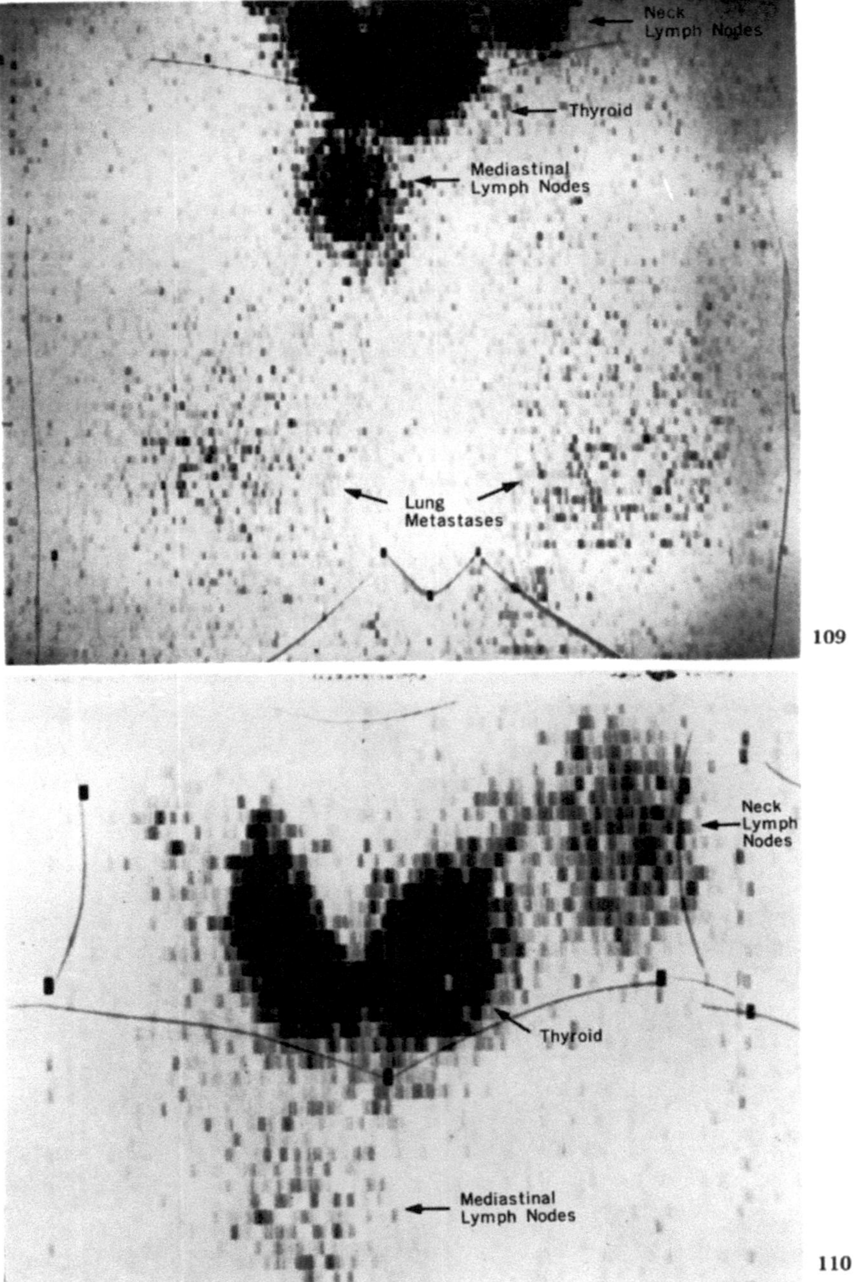

Fig. 109, 110 Scintiscanning of the neck and chest with radioiodine. Radioiodine was taken up by lymph node metastases in both jugular chains and the right upper mediastinum, and also by the metastatic lesions in the lungs.

Case 14. Incidentally Discovered Round, Calcified Thyroid Nodule: Follicular Carcinoma (Group VII in Table 13)

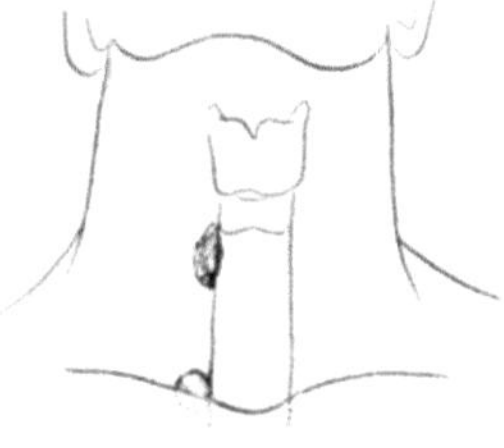

Fig. 111

T. D., 48-year-old woman came to the hospital in June, 1971, for consultation regarding her daughter's swollen thyroid, which proved to be a simple diffuse goiter. The patient herself did not have any complaints, but was incidentally found to have firm mass, fixed to the trachea, about 1 cm in diameter, in the right lobe of the thyroid (Fig. 111).

Roentgenograms of the neck revealed no calcification in the palpated mass, but a round calcified nodule approximately 1 cm in diameter was found on the film at the level of the clavicle (Fig. 112). It was only after roentgenograpihc study thatthe upper portion of this deeply situated nodule could be palpated on swallowing.

The right lobe of the thyroid was removed and lymph nodes were dissected from the right paratracheal region (Fig. 113). Pathological examination showed that the mass first noted on palpation was due to a focal type of autoimmune thyroiditis, and the calcified nodule at the lower pole was a follicular carcinoma with a thick fibrous calcified capsule (Figs. 114, 115). Microscopically there was no evidence of lymph node metastasis.

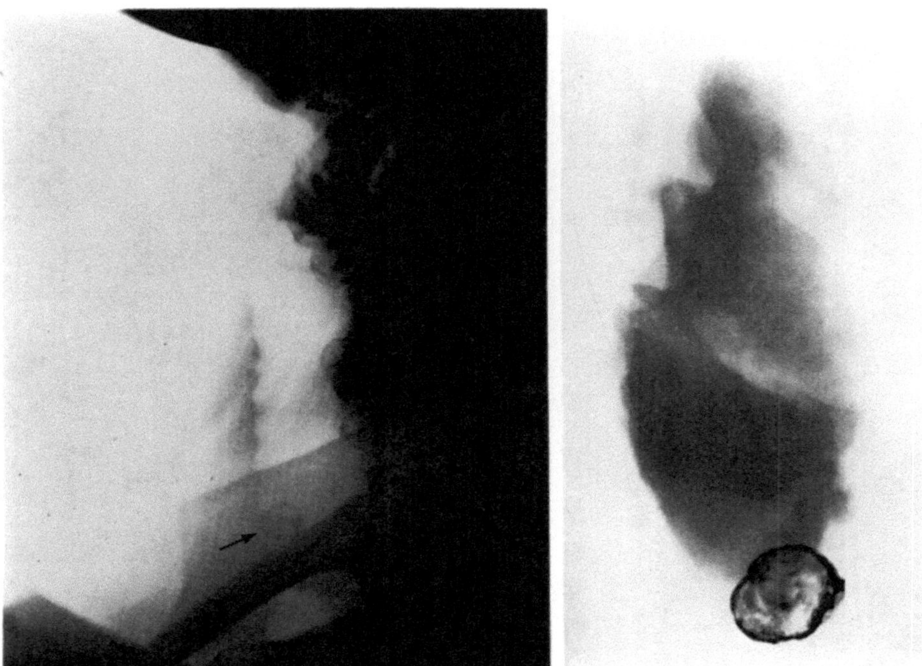

Fig. 112 Lateral soft tissue roentgenogram of the neck. A calcified nodule is seen at the level of the clavicle (arrow).

Fig. 113 Roentgenogram of the removed right thyroid lobe. The calcified nodule is in the lower pole of the lobe.

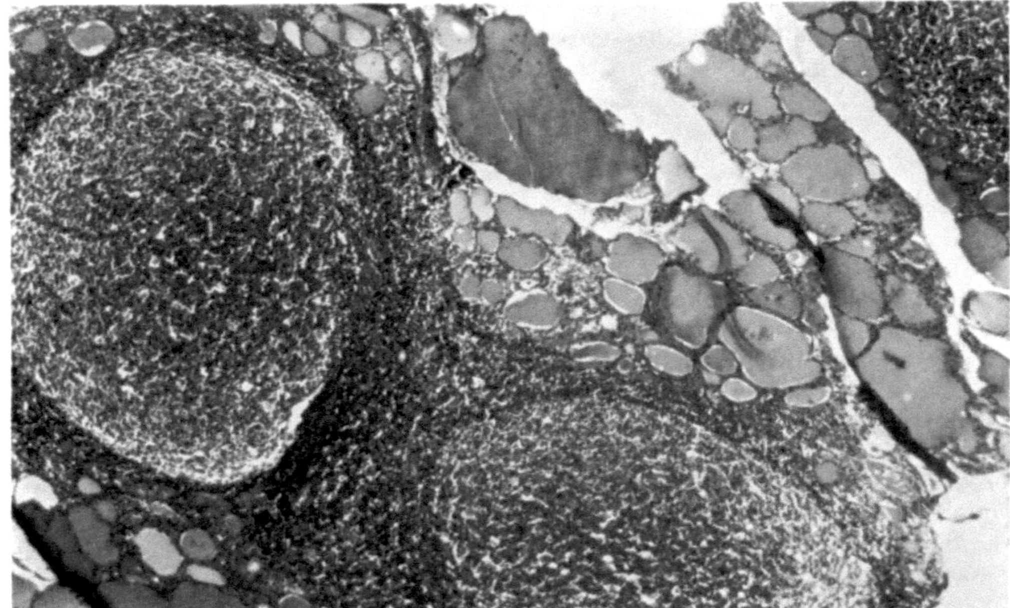

Fig. 114   Histologic section of the lesion in the superior portion of the right lobe of the thyroid palpated preoperatively as a firm mass.   The findings are focal lymphocytic thyroiditis with lymph follicle formation.   (H & E, × 100)

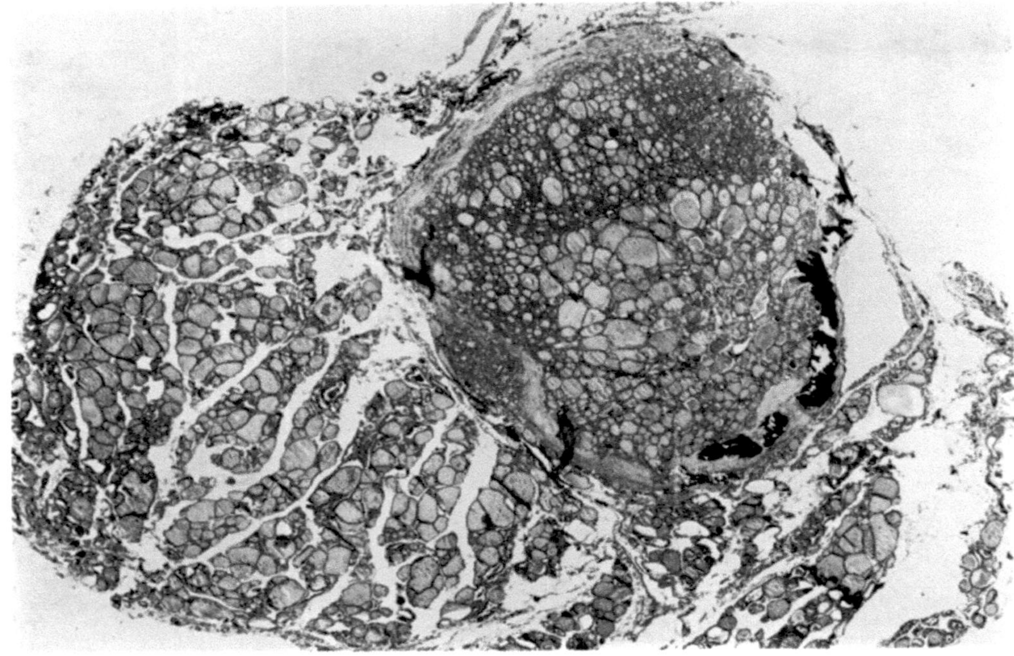

Fig. 115   Photomicrograph of the calcified nodule. Histologically it is a follicular carcinoma with thick fibrous capsule containing the calcium depositions.   (H & E, × 10)

Case 15.   Papillary Carcinoma of the Thyroid Detected by
Lymph Node Involvement (Group III in Table13)

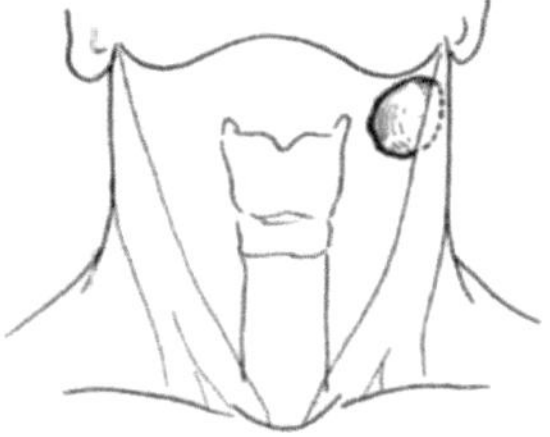

Fig. 116

T. D., a 61-year-old woman visited the hopital in October, 1970, complaining of a lump at the left submaxillary region.   She had been aware of the mass for about 10 years but recently it began to enlarge rapidly.

Examination revealed a smooth but hard, non-mobile, 3 cm mass in the left submaxillary area (Fig. 116).   Lymph node involvement by cancer of unknown origin was suspected, but physical examination was normal including the oropharynx, thyroid and major salivery glands.   An open biopsy was performed.   Histologic sections revealed lymph nodes affected by metastatic papillary carcinoma of the thyroid.

After the biopsy, the thyroid gland was re-examined carefully, but no tumor was palpated.   Roentgenograms of the neck demonstrated a round calcific deposit of about 3 mm in diameter (Fig. 117).

At the time of operation, a tumor with a calcified capsule was found in the middle of the left lobe, and also another occult tumor measuring a few millimeters in diameter was discovered at the upper pole of the left lobe (Fig. 118).   Subtotal thyroidectomy and modified neck dissection were carried out.   On histologic sections, both of the thyroid tumors proved to be carcinomas; the upper one showed a predominantly papillary growth (Fig. 119), and the lower one had a follicular pattern surrounded by a thick fibrous capsule with calcium deposits (Fig. 120).   There were several lymph nodes containing metastatic lesions in the left jugular chain.

Postoperative course was uneventful.

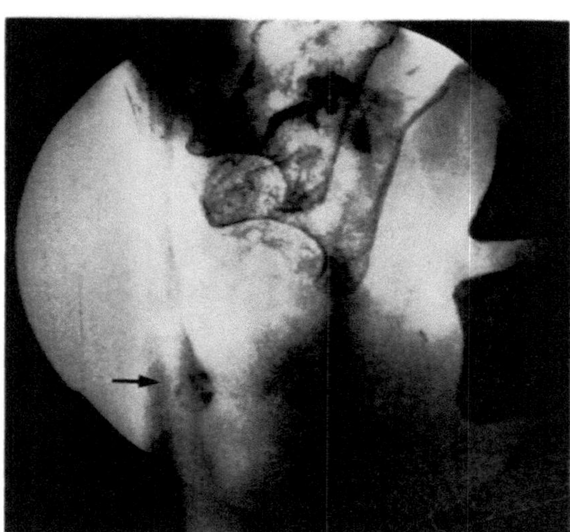

Fig. 117   Spot-tangential view showing a very
small calcified nodule (arrow).

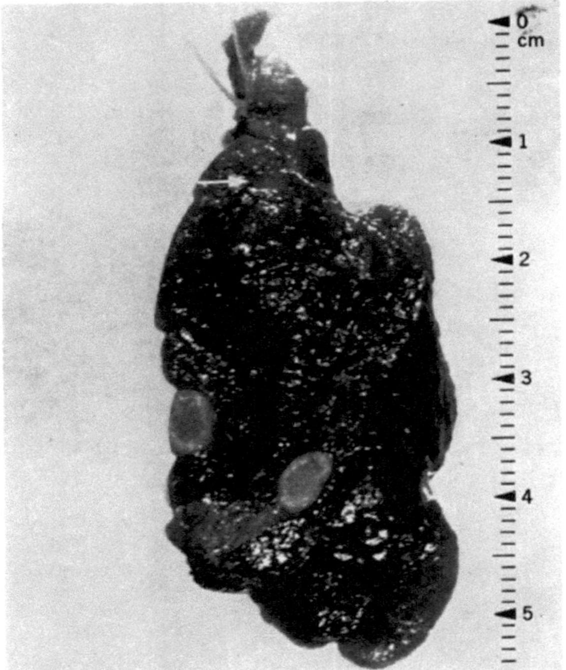

Fig. 118 Cut surface of the left lobe of the thyroid. In addition to a well-encapsulated, calcified nodule, there is an occult carcinoma in the upper pole of the lobe (arrow).

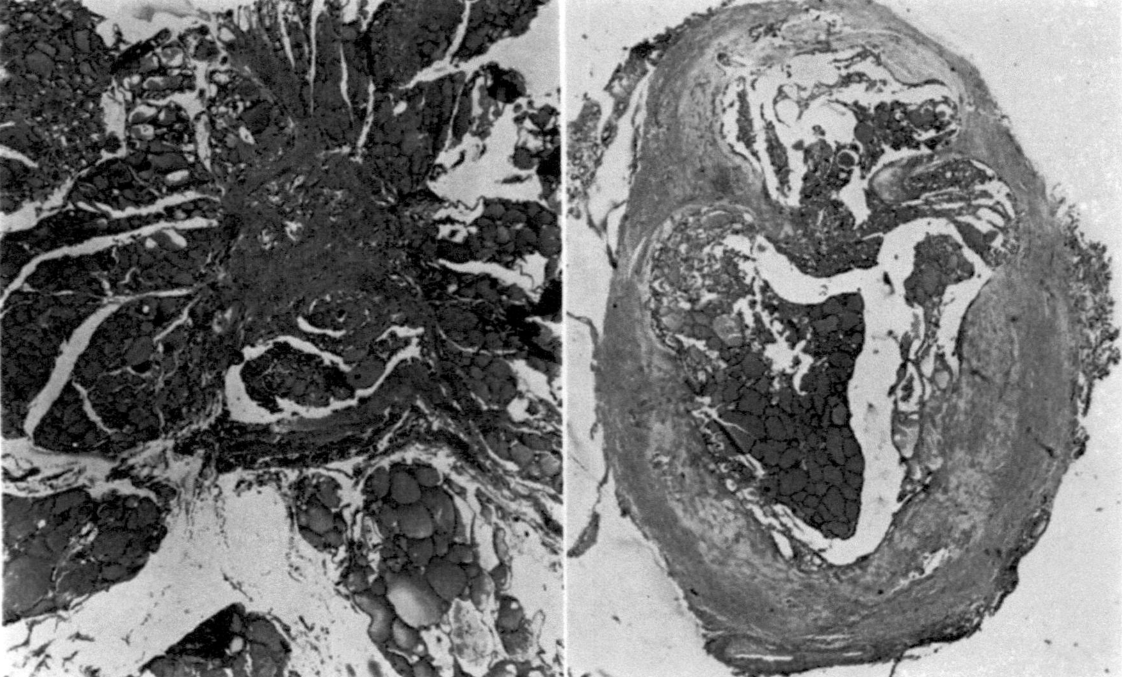

Fig. 119 Microscopic appearance of the 3 mm occult papillary carcinoma located in the upper pole. (H & E, × 15)

Fig. 120 Photomicrograph of the tumor located in the mid portion of the lobe. Histologically it is diagnosed as papillary carcinoma with a predominantly follicular pattern. Marked calcification occurred in the fibrous capsule. (H & E, × 15)

Case 16. Papillary Carcinoma of the Thyroid Detected Due to Recurrent Laryngeal Nerve Palsy (Classified in Group III in Table 13 because of non-palpable primary tumor)

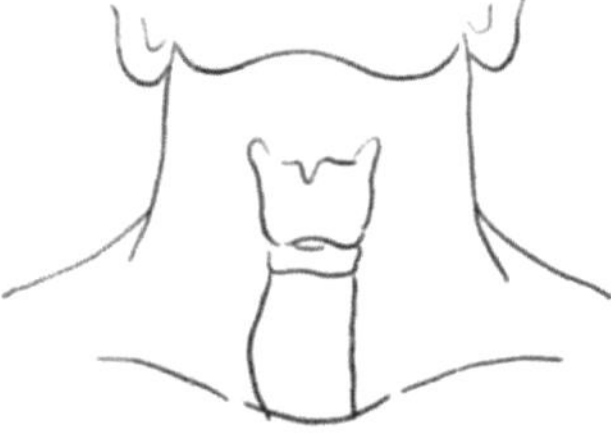

Fig. 121

S. K., a 61-year-old man was referred to us by an otolaryngologist for an evaluation of a thyroid lesion as a probable cause of the recurrent nerve palsy on the left side in September, 1970. The patient first noticed hoarseness about five years previously, and one month prior to the visit he became aphonic temporarily after an operation for the urinary bladder tumor performed under endotracheal anesthesia.

Examination revealed no tumor mass along the course of the left recurrent nerve. A routine roentgenogram of the neck disclosed irregular compression of the trachea on the affected side (Fig. 122). Soft tissue roentgenogram showed a small coarse calcific deposit (Fig. 123). From these results, an occult carcinoma of the thyroid was strongly suspected.

At operation, a papillary carcinoma 8 mm in diameter was found with a metastatic lesion to one paratracheal lymph node, both of which had invaded the trachea and the recurrent laryngeal nerve was encased within the tumor. In order to remove the cancer completely, a 1 × 1.5 cm area of the cartilage layer of the trachea where the tumor was fixed was resected and the recurrent nerve had to be sacrificed (Fig. 124). Subtotal thyroidectomy and modified neck dissection on the affected side were carried out.

The patient has been doing well except for a residual hoarseness.

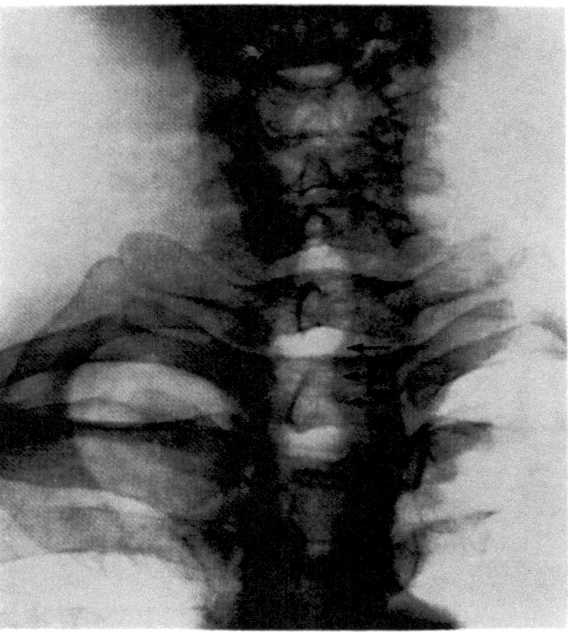

Fig. 122 Antero-posterior roentgenogram of the neck. The trachea is displaced to the right and its left wall is indented.

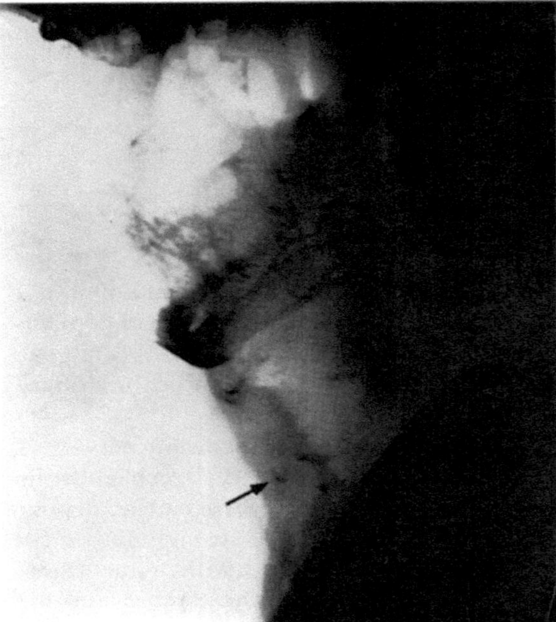

Fig. 123 Lateral soft tissue roentgenogram of the neck. In addition to the calcified tracheal rings, a coarse punctate calcific deposit is seen anterior to the trachea (arrow).

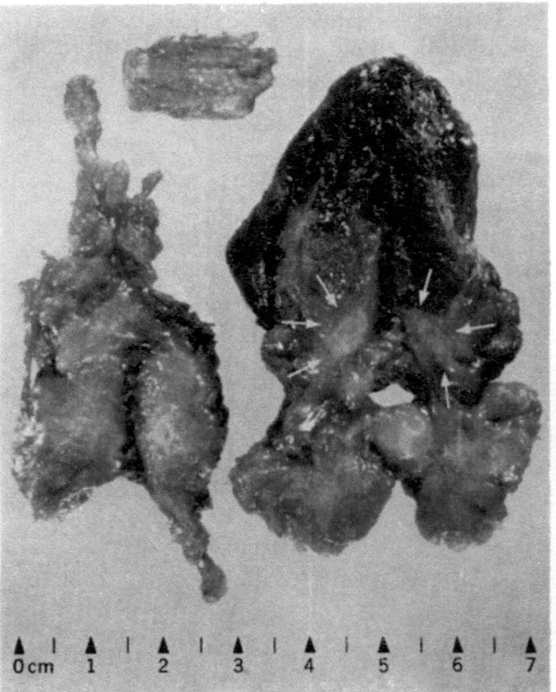

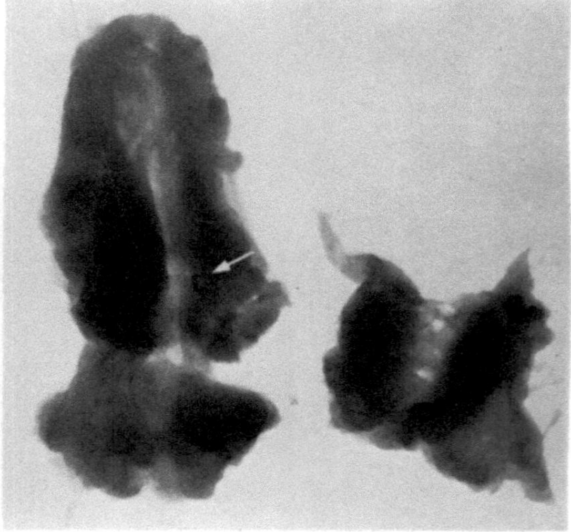

Fig. 124 Cut surface of the resected specimens. Right: left lobe of the thyroid and paratracheal lymph nodes. A 8 × 4 mm carcinoma in the lower pole of the thyroid (arrows) and involved nodes. Left: dissected specimen from the left jugular region, showing lymph nodes involved by metastases. Upper: removed cartilage layer of the trachea, to which the primary cancer was firmly fixed.

Fig. 125 Specimen roentgenogram showing coarse calcific deposits and a few psammomatous shadows at the site of primary cancer.

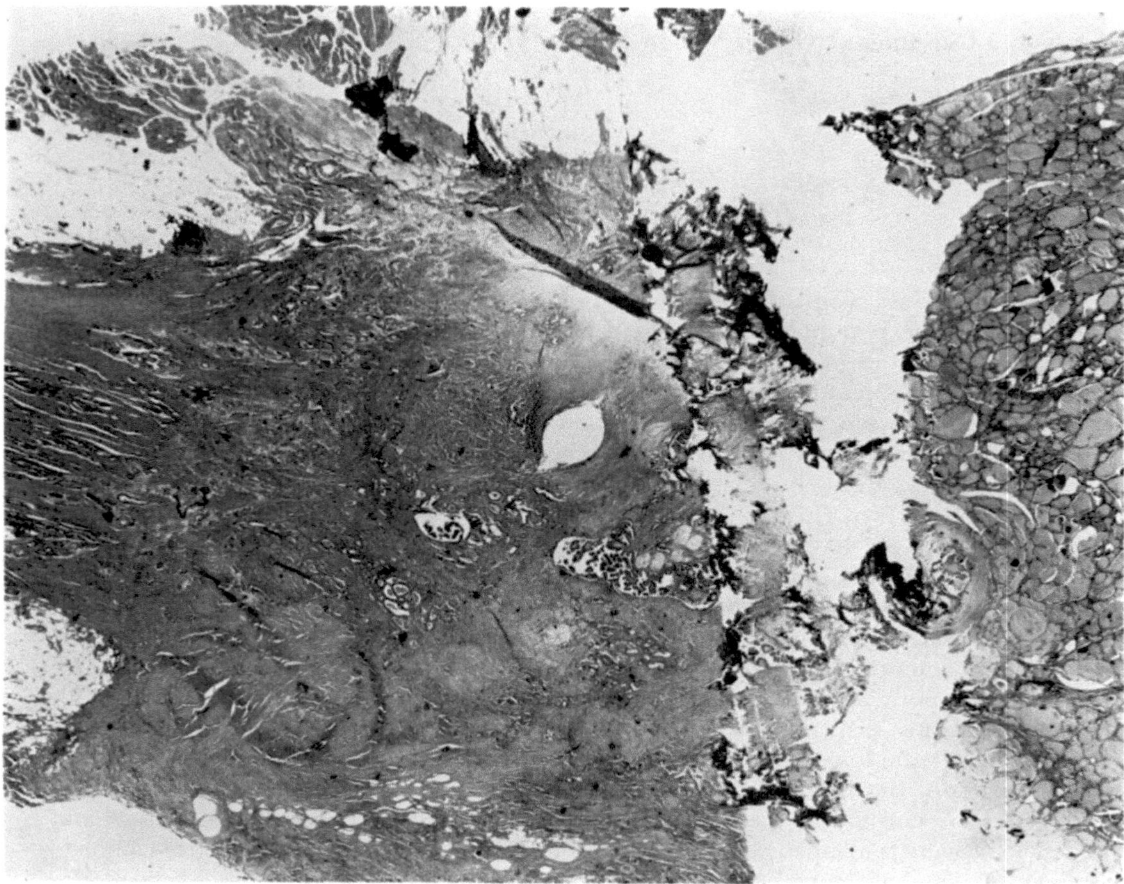

Fig. 126 Photomicrograph of specimen, showing papillary carcinoma of the thyroid with abundant fibrous stroma. The section was damaged on cutting through the densely calcified area. (H & E, × 7)

Case 17.   Graves' Disease Associated with a Small Papillary
Carcinoma (Group VII in Table 13)

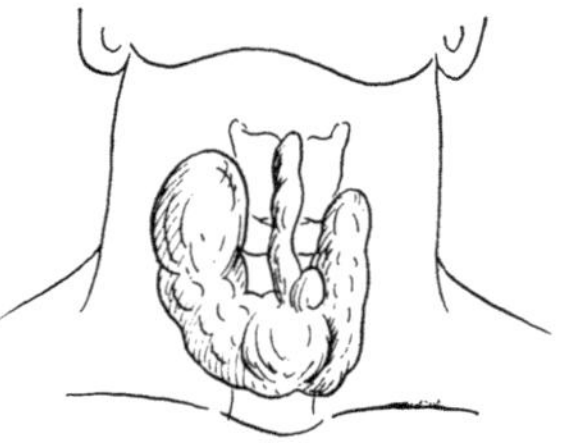

Fig. 127

T. G., a 50-year-old woman visited the hospital in November, 1970, because of a diffuse, firm goiter.   One year previously she had palpitation, weight loss and heat intolerance, and was diagnosed as having Graves' disease at another hospital.   She had been treated medically, but one month prior to her visit she had stopped taking her medications.

On examination, the patient was a well-nourished woman without apparent symptoms of thyrotoxicosis except for a slight hand tremor.   Exophthalmos was not present.   The thyroid gland was diffusely enlarged to almost three times normal size and felt grossly nodular and very firm (Fig. 127). ^{131}I thyroid uptake at 24 hours was 79.5%, BMR +36% and T_3 RSU 40.2%.   Thyroid suppression test carried out after 75 μg of triiodothyronine daily for seven days showed ^{131}I uptake at 24 hours of 11%.   Thyroid scintigram showed several areas of low radioiodine uptake.   Roentgenogram of the neck revealed a densely calcified nodule of about 1×0.5 cm adjacent to the cricoid cartilage anteriorly and another punctate calcific deposite lower in the thyroid gland (Fig. 128).   From these results, a toxic nodular goiter was suspected first, but later Graves' disease associated with thyroid neoplasms, probably malignant, was thought to be more likely, and surgery was performed after the toxic state was suppressed by propylthiouracil.

At operation, the thyroid was diffusely enlarged with an unusually firm consistency and a hard 1.5 cm nodule (carcinoma) was found at the area between the isthmus and the left lobe, which invaded the trachea.   Subtotal thyroidectomy including a complete removal of the carcinoma was performed.   Lymph nodes were removed from the paratracheal regions bilaterally.

Review of the specimen roentgenogram and the microscopic sections showed two areas of calcium deposition; one was in the carcinoma (Fig. 129) and the other was in the fibrous scar tissue within the right lobe whose cause was not determined.   The conclusive diagnosis was Graves' disease associated with papillary carcinoma of the thyroid.

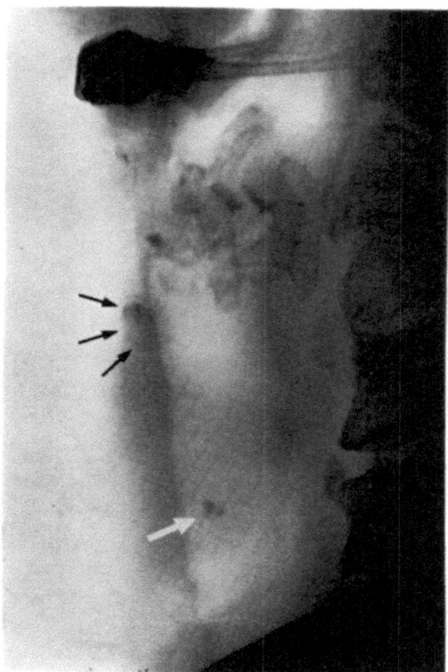

Fig. 128 Lateral soft tissue roentgenogram of the neck, showing a round calcified nodule (black arrows) anterior to and slightly below the cricoid cartilage (arrow) and a punctate calcific deposit (white arrow) in the lower region of the neck.

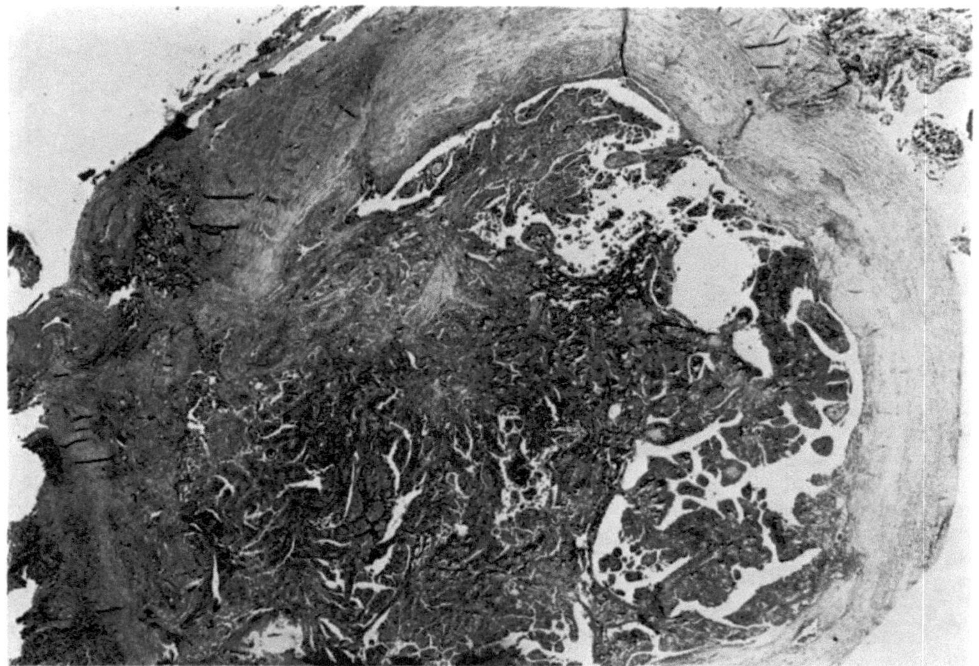

Fig. 129 Microscopic section of papillary carcinoma of the thyroid, which was in the upper part of the isthmus. The tumor capsule is densely calcified. (H & E, × 7).

Case 18. Hashimoto's Disease Associated with Thyroid
Carcinoma (Group VII in Table 13)

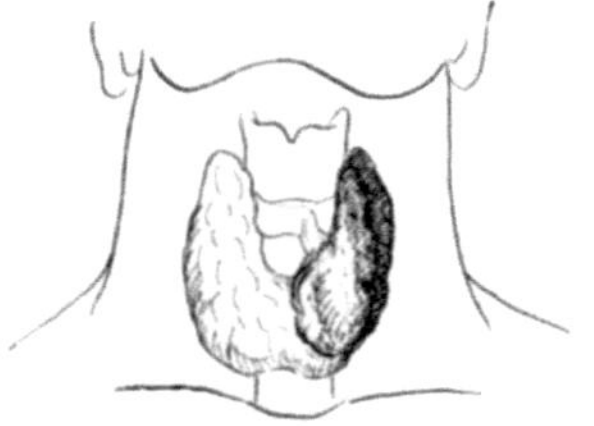

Fig. 130

S. M., a 77-year-old woman was referred to us in March, 1971, by a physician because of
a nodular mass in a diffuse, firm goiter.   The patient first noticed the painless swelling of
her thyroid two years previously and was diagnosed as having Hashimoto's disease.   She
began to notice difficulty in swallowing five months prior to the visit.

Examination revealed the thyroid gland to be firm and diffusely enlarged.   Autoimmune thyroiditis was suspected, but the upper two thirds of the left lobe was rather hard
and irregular, arousing suspicion of a malignant tumor (Fig. 130).   Roentgenograms of
the neck showed a massive calcification at the upper portion of the left lobe (Fig. 131).
Laryngoscopic examination revealed left vocal cord paralysis.   Barium swallow demonstrated marked narrowing over a three centimeter length (Fig. 132).   These findings
indicated the presence of carcinoma of the thyroid in association with Hashimoto's disease.

Since the patient was old and malnourished with a body weight of only 25 kg, she has
been treated conservatively with 50 to 75 mg of desiccated thyroid daily.

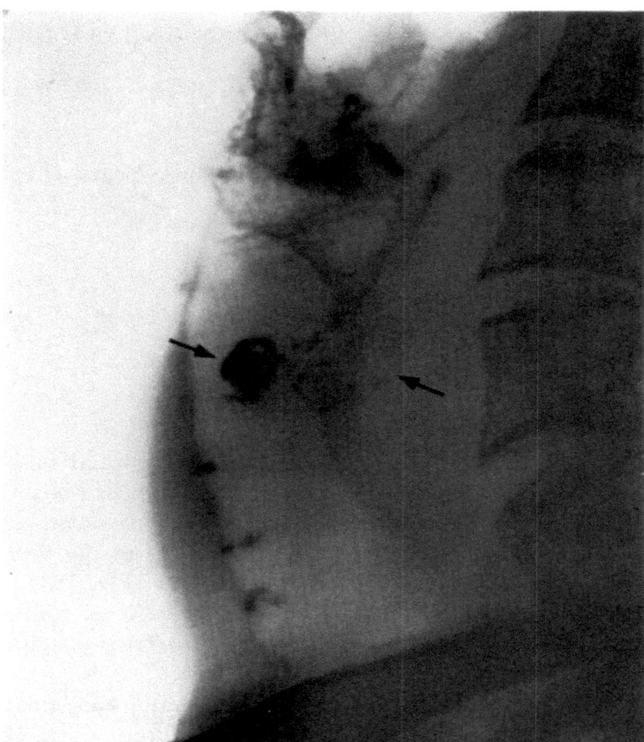

Fig. 131 Lateral soft tissue roentgenogram of the neck, showing two massive calcifications, one more densely calcified than the other. The trachea is compressed from behind.

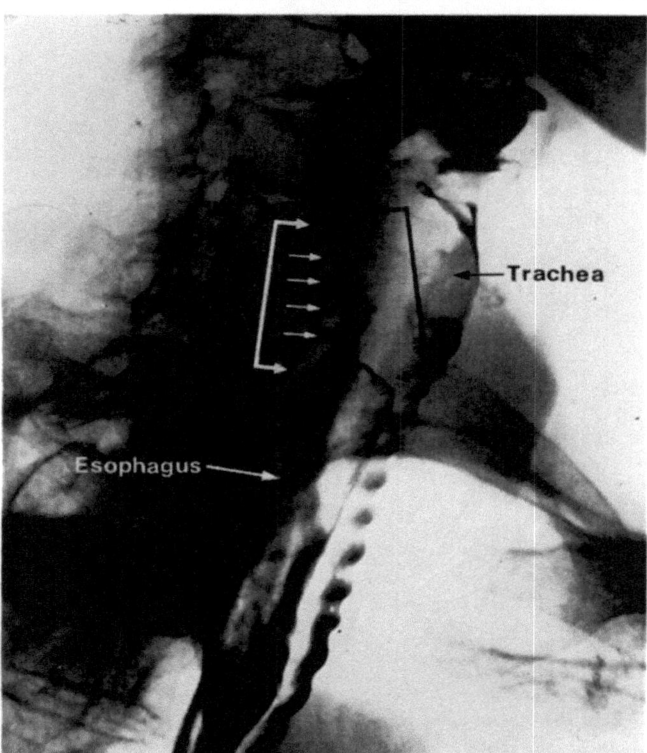

Fig. 132 Barium swallow showed a marked constriction of the esophagus due to the invasive growth of the thyroid cancer. Since the patient had the left recurrent nerve palsy, a small amount of barium entered into the larynx and trachea.

III. BENIGN NODULES PRESENTING COARSE CALCIFICATIONS ON NECK ROENTGENOGRAMS

Case 19. Adenomatous Goiter of Three Years' Duration

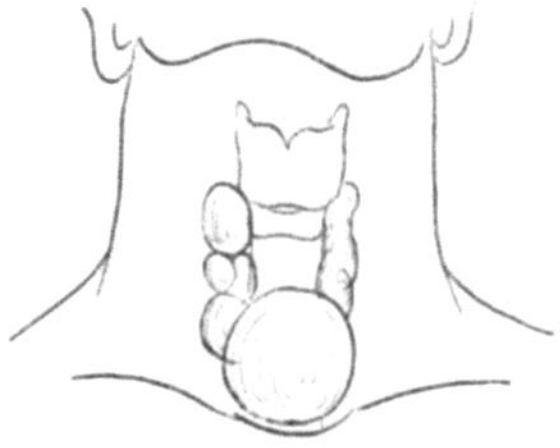

Fig. 133

S. S., a 35-year-old woman visited the hospital in November, 1970, complaining of a lump in the middle of her anterior neck of three years' duration.   Eight months previously she noted a sudden enlargement of the nodule accompanied by fever and local tenderness.

Examination revealed multiple nodules in the thyroid.   The largest one was located in the isthmus and was 2 cm in diameter (Fig. 133).   Roentgenograms of the neck presented many coarse calcifications of various configulations (Fig. 134).   An adenomatous goiter was suspected, but an associated occult carcinoma of the thyroid could not be ruled out.

At the time of operation, only adenomatous nodules were found and were removed without complication (Fig. 136).   She has been given 100 mg of desiccated thyroid daily following surgery.

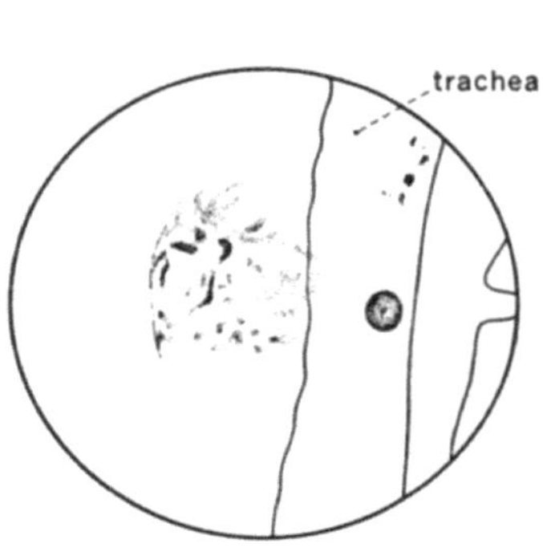

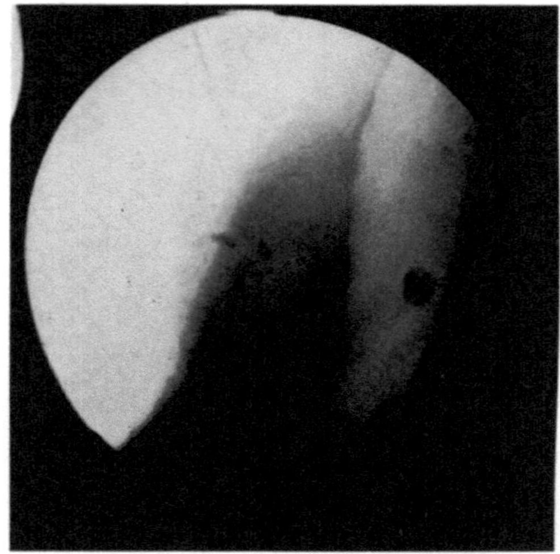

Fig. 134   Spot-tangential views of the neck, showing several coarse calcifications of various configurations.   This is the common roentgenographic appearance in adenomatous goiter.

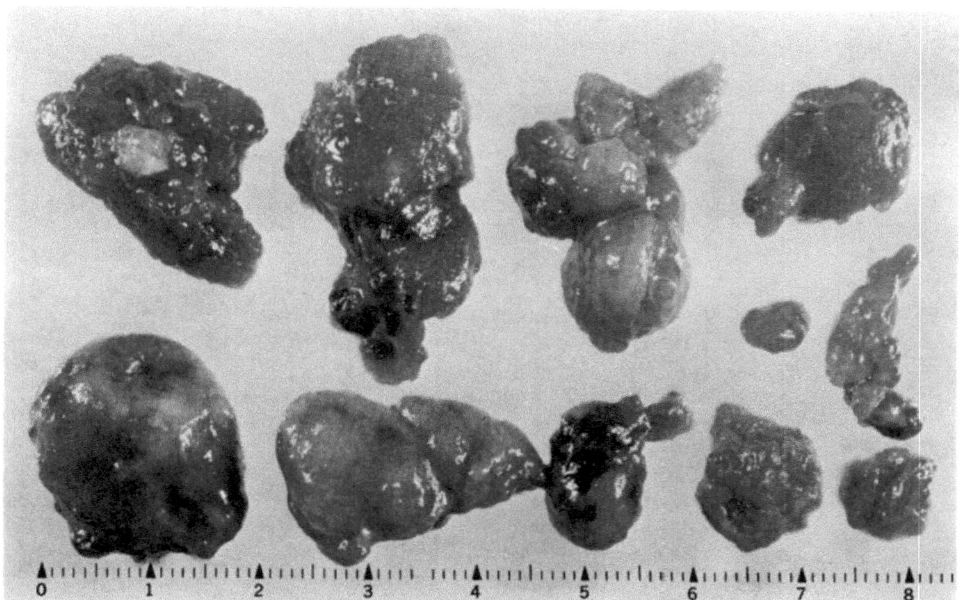

Fig. 135   Surgically removed specimens.

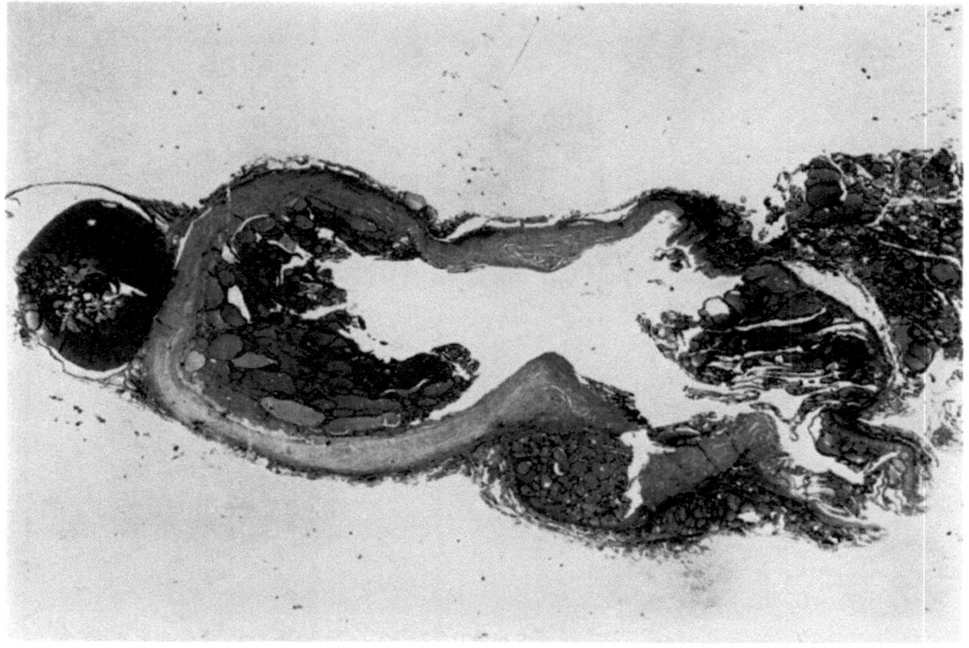

Fig. 136   Photomicrograph of specimen.   Coarse calcification occurred within the thick fibrous capsule. (H & E, × 7)

Case 20. Another Example of Adenomatous Goiter that Presented a Variety of Coarse Calcifications on Neck X-Rays

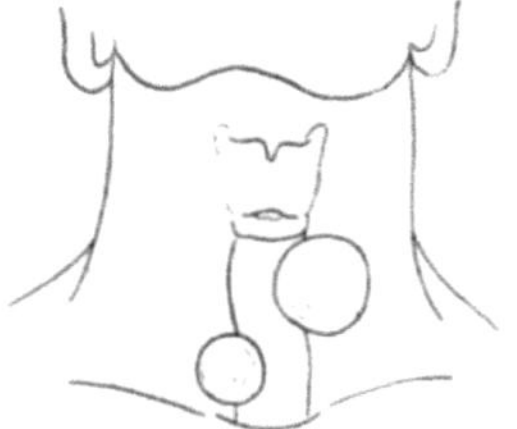

Fig. 137

A. N., a 56-year-old housewife was admitted to the hospital in April, 1970, for surgical removal of thyroid nodules which were noticed two months previously.

Examination revealed two thyroid nodules of 1 and 2 cm in diameter respectively, both of which were round and easily movable (Fig. 137). Soft tissue roentgenograms showed a round calcified nodule and irregular punctate calcium deposits (Fig. 138). The diagnostic impression was an adenomatous goiter.

At operation, total of four nodules were found in the thyroid and all were removed. Microscopically they were confirmed to be benign adenomatous nodules (Fig. 139). Post-operative course was uneventful.

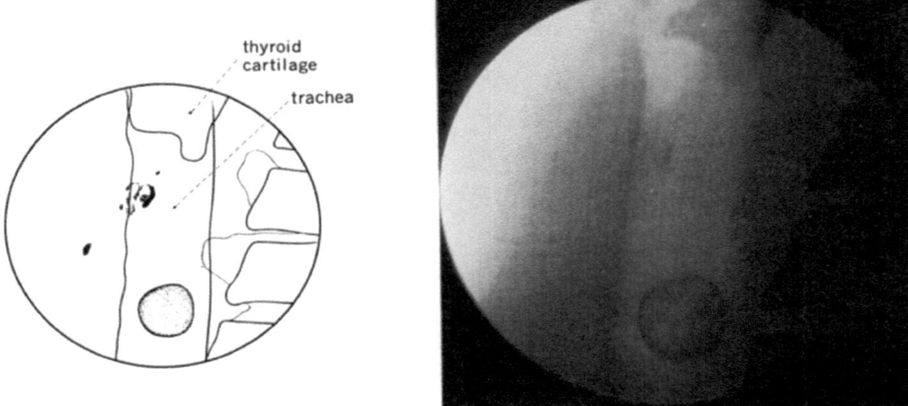

Fig. 138 Spot-tangential view of soft tissue roentgenogram, showing a round calcified nodule and several coarse calcific deposits.

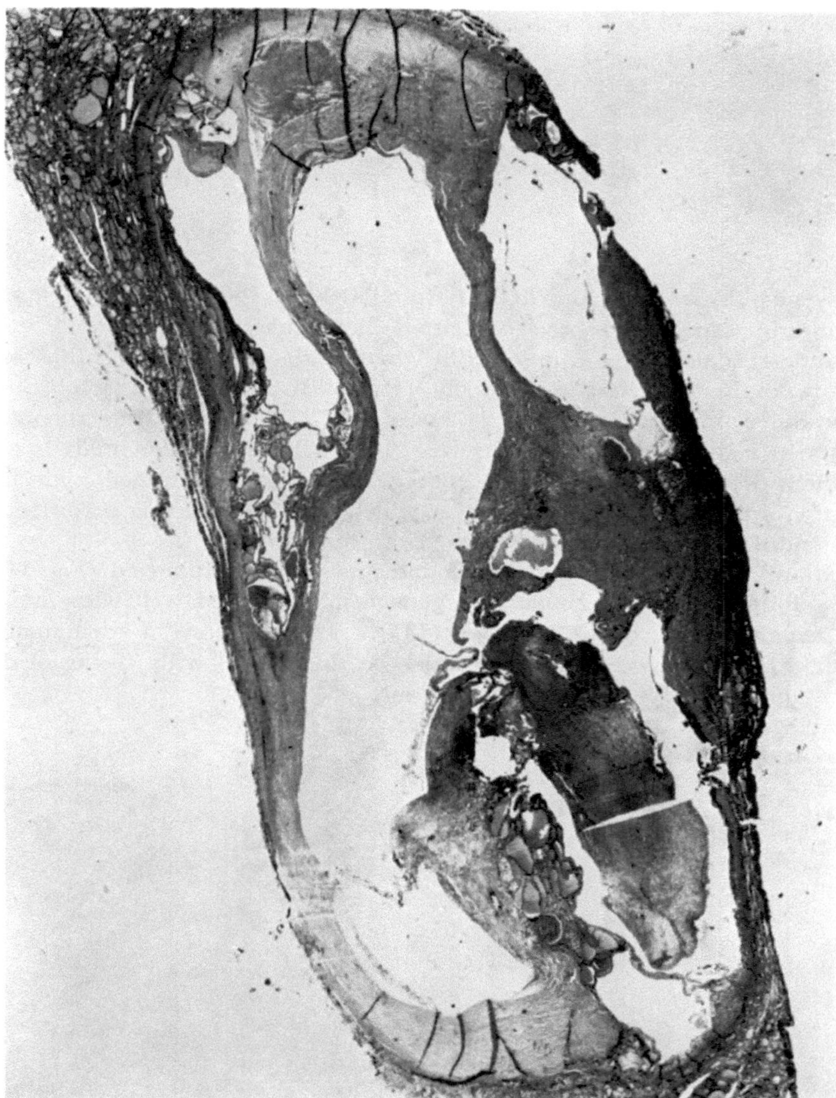

Fig. 139 Histologic section of one of the nodules, showing a thick fibrous, calcified capsule and cystic degeneration of the nodule. (H & E, × 7)

Case 21. Adenomatous Goiter of Six Years' Duration

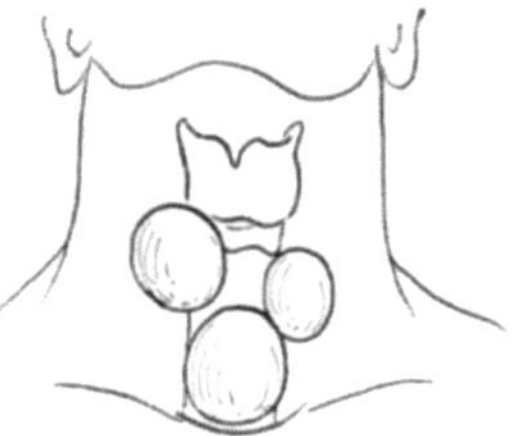

Fig. 140

K. T., a 22-year-old man first came to the hospital in May, 1969, because of painless swelling in the anterior aspect of the neck, which was noticed six years previously.

Examination revealed three nodules in the thyroid gland, readily movable, round and 3, 3 and 2.5 cm in diameter, respectively (Fig. 140). BMR was$+10\%$, T_3 RSU was 32% and ^{131}I thyroid uptake at 24 hours was 21%. Soft tissue roentgenograms revealed several coarse calcium deposits (Fig. 141). Thus an adenomatous goiter was suspected clinically. The patient had epilepsy and was maintained with 100 mg of desiccated thyroid daily for nine months, at which time surgery was performed because the thyroid nodules had enlarged despite medical treatment.

At operation, numerous nodules were found and all were removed (Fig. 142). The calcifications found on the specimen roentgenogram correlated well with those on pre-operative roentgenograms of the neck (Fig. 143). The diagnosis of adenomatous goiter was confirmed by histologic study. He has been doing well with 75 mg of desiccated thyroid daily up to now.

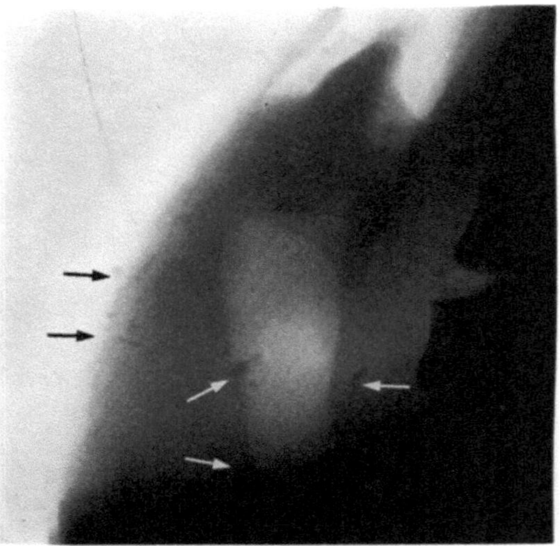

Fig. 141 Lateral view of the neck showing calcifications in punctate and curvilinear patterns.

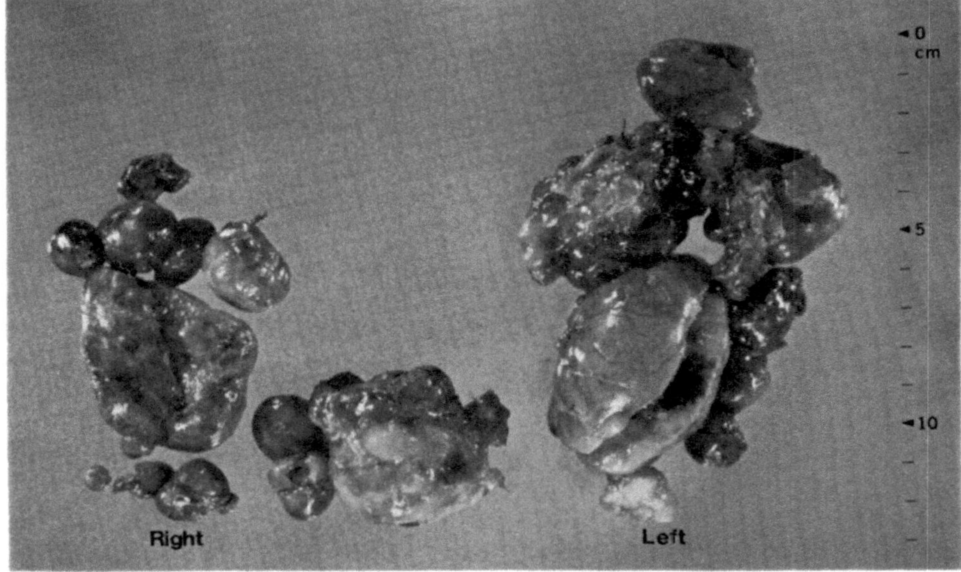

Fig. 142 Surgically removed specimens.

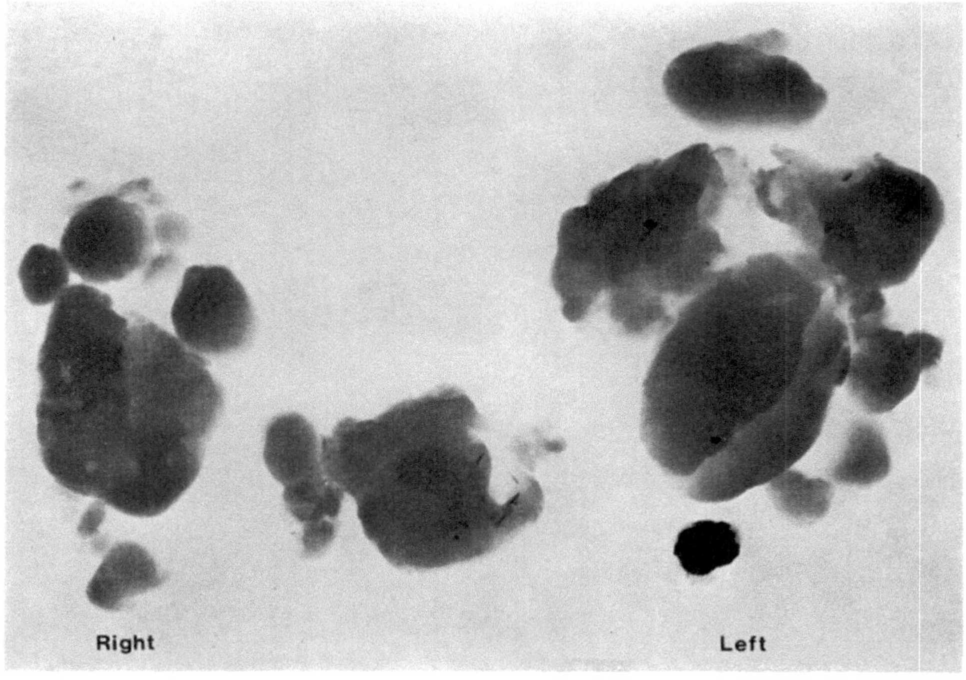

Fig. 143 Roentgenogram of the specimens.

Case 22.   A Large Adenoma of Eight Years' Duration

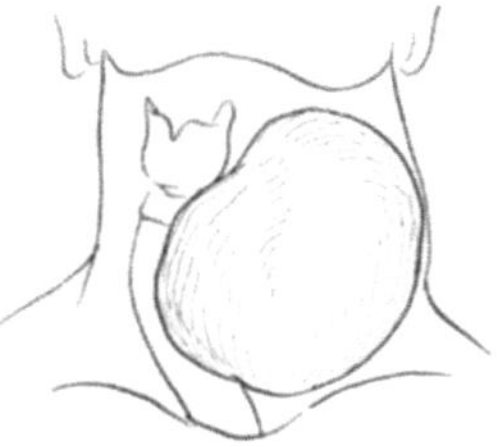

Fig. 144

M. T., a 62-year-old woman visited the hospital in June, 1971, with a large tumor in the neck of eight years' duration.   The tumor increased in size gradually without causing any compression symptoms.

Examination revealed a soft, 9×10 cm fluctuant nodule in the neck.   The trachea was deviated to the right by the tumor (Fig. 144).   Roentgenograms of the neck showed several coarse calcium deposits (Fig. 145).   Ultrasonic scanning disclosed the tumor to be cystic and 25 ml of clear fluid was aspirated.

At surgery, the left lobe of the thyroid including the tumor was easily removed.   It was a colloid adenoma with a large cystic cavity, the wall of which contained most of the calcifications (Figs. 146, 147).

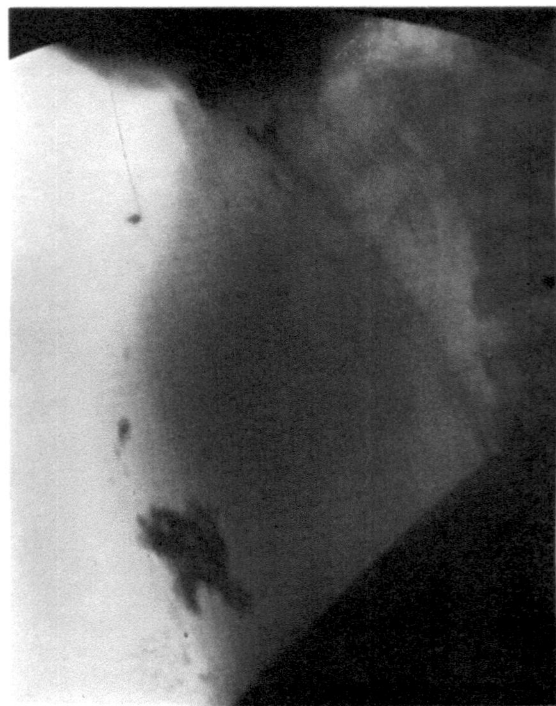

Fig. 145   Lateral view of the neck, showing a large area of amorphous calcification and several small calcific deposits.

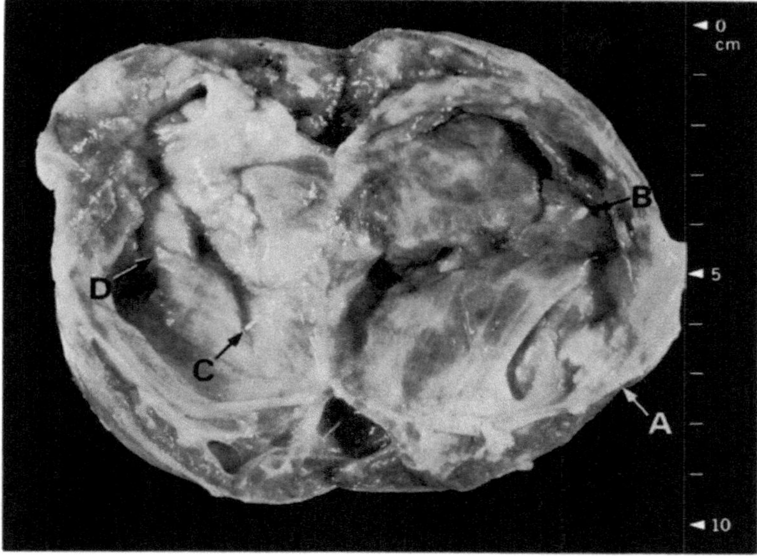

Fig. 146 Cut surface of the left thyroid lobe.   The nodule has a large cystic cavity and most of the calcified flecks were found in the cyst wall.

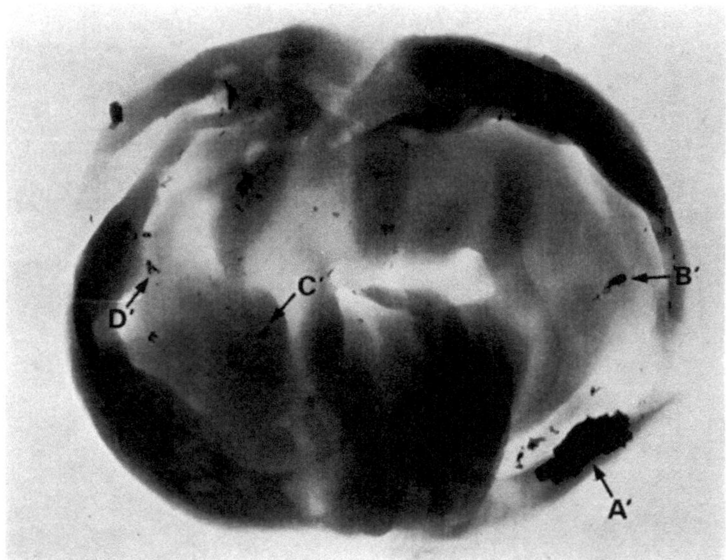

Fig. 147 Roentgenogram of the specimen.

Case 23.   A Huge Adenoma of 38 Years' Duration

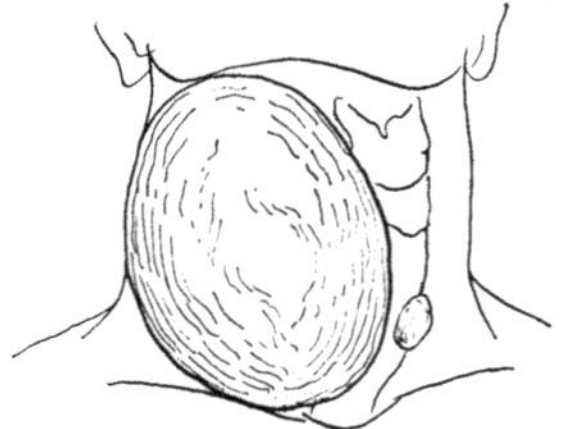

Fig. 148

Y. K., a 67-year-old woman came to our hospital in January, 1971, with a huge tumor in the neck, which was first noticed 38 years previously and had gradually increased in size. She had irradiation therapy for the tumor 15 years previously.

The patient was clinically euthyroid.   The neck mass measured 10 cm in diameter and deviated the trachea to the left (Fig. 148).   The ultrasonic examination revealed the tumor to be a solid one.   Roentgenograms of the neck showed coarse and amorphous calcifications (Figs. 149, 150, 151).   No abnormal lymph node swelling was noted in the neck.

A right lobectomy was performed including the tumor.   Pathological examination revealed a benign tubular adenoma of the thyroid.   Massive deposits of calcium were found in the fibrous capsule of the tumor and in the trabeculae within the tumor (Fig. 152).

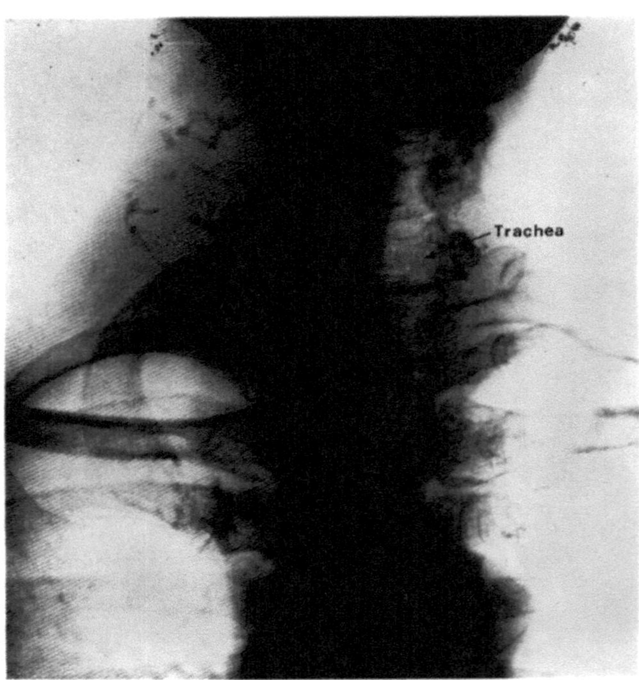

Fig. 149 Standard antero-posterior view of the neck, showing deviation and compression of the trachea toward the left and multiple calcific shadows of amorphous and curvilinear configulations within the tumor.

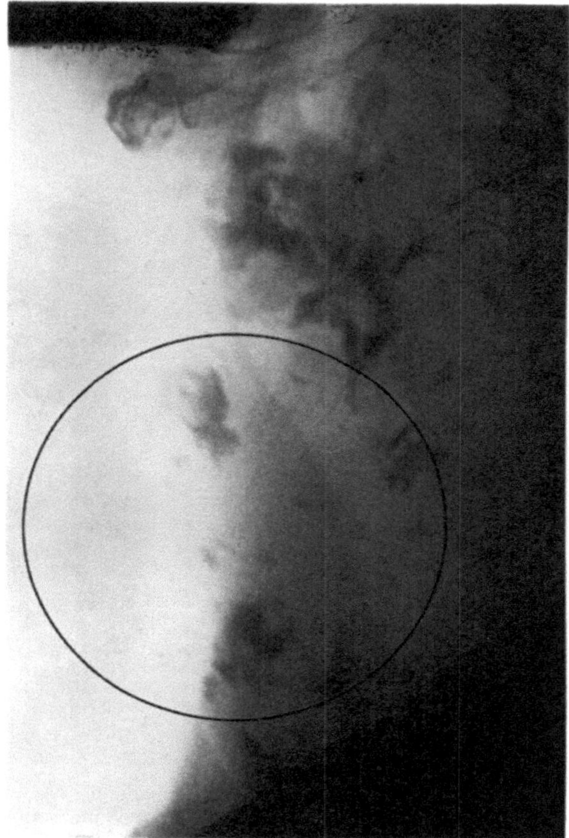

Fig. 150 Lateral view.

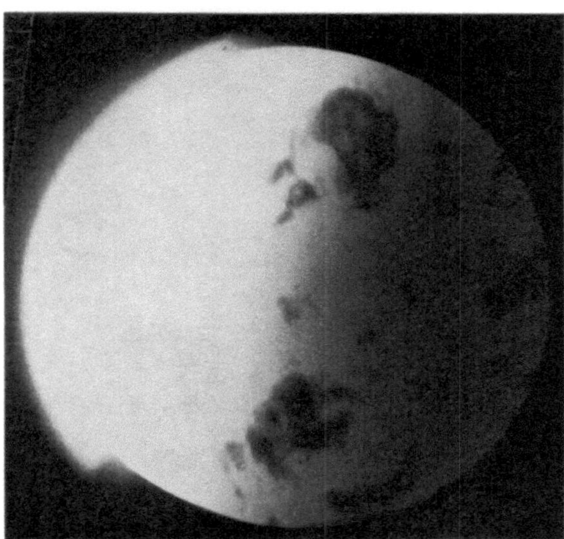

Fig. 151 Spot-tangential view, showing the same area as encircled on the lateral view. Coarse calcifications of various configulations are more clearly outlined on this view.

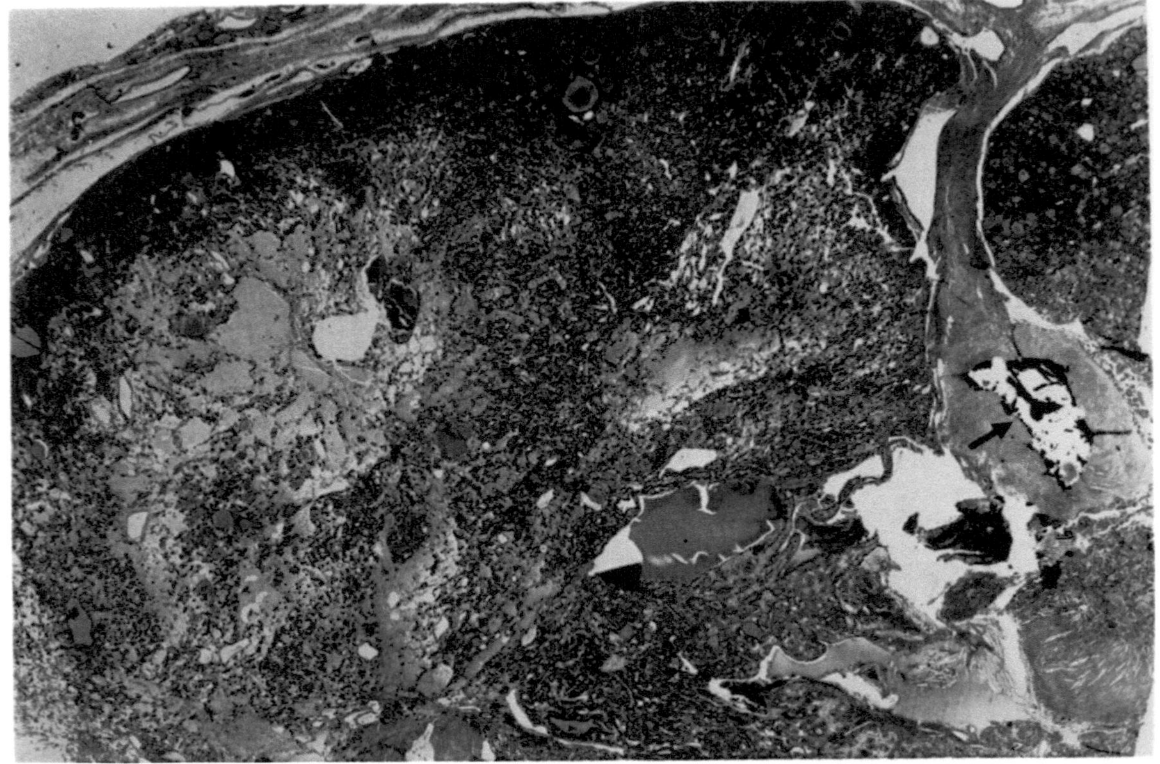

Fig. 152 Microscopic section of the nodule. A microfollicular adenoma of the thyroid with fibrous trabecula, in which massive calcium deposition occurred. (H & E, × 7)

Case 24. Enormous Nodules Occupying Almost the Entire
Anterior Part of the Neck

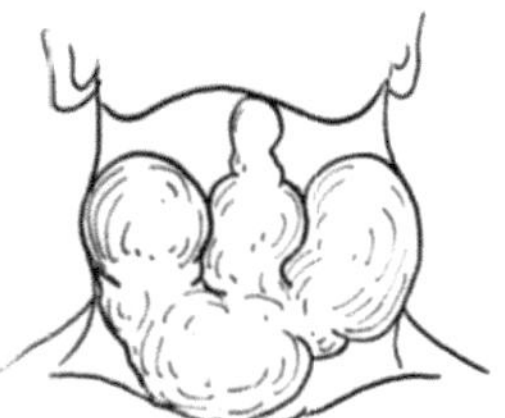

Fig. 153

S. O., a 56-year-old woman was admitted to the Hospital of Institute of Medical Science, University of Tokyo, in August, 1971, because of a marked enlargement of the neck of 35 years' duration.

On examination, she was found to have a huge nodular tumor. The mass occupied almost the entire anterior part of the neck, and the common carotid arteries were palpated lateral to the outer margins of the tumor bilaterally (Fig. 153). Initially controversy arose as to the origin and nature of this enormous tumor, including the possibility of dermoid cyst, but its paratracheal location and upward movement on swallowing suggested that it was most likely of thyroid origin. Observation of multiple cold nodules on the thyroid scintigram gave us definitive information as to the thyroid origin of the tumor. ^{131}I thyroidal uptake at 24 hours was 25.5%, T_3 RSU 25.6% and T_4 9.5 μg per 100 ml. Standard roentgenograms of the neck revealed coarse calcium deposits in several of the nodules (Figs. 154, 155).

Subtotal thyroidectomy was performed with removal of all of the nodules (Fig. 156). Microscopically the nodules showed the histological appearance of adenomatous goiter (Fig. 157). Postoperative course was uneventful. She has been given desiccated thyroid, 75 mg daily.

 CASE REPORTS

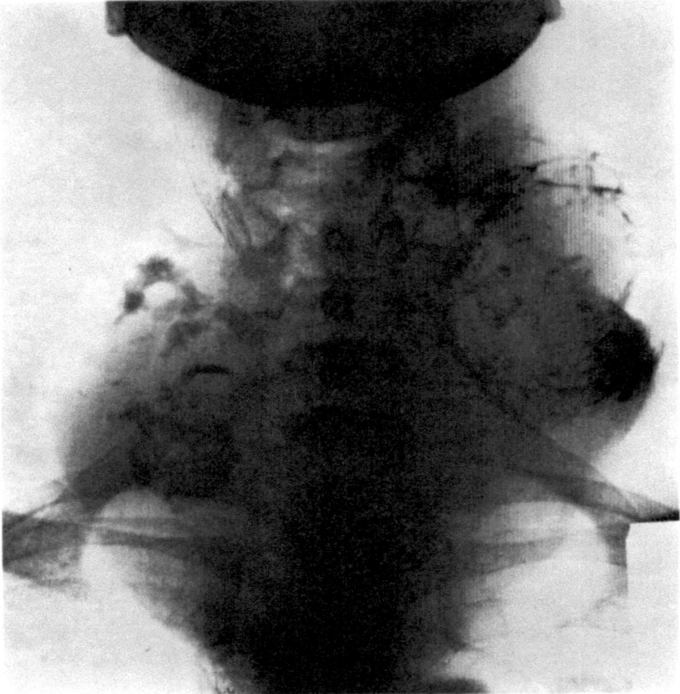

Fig. 154 Standard antero-posterior view of the neck. The outline of the neck tumor is seen as a dense mass. The massive calcifications seen on the right are amorphous and those seen in the left upper neck have a circular pattern.

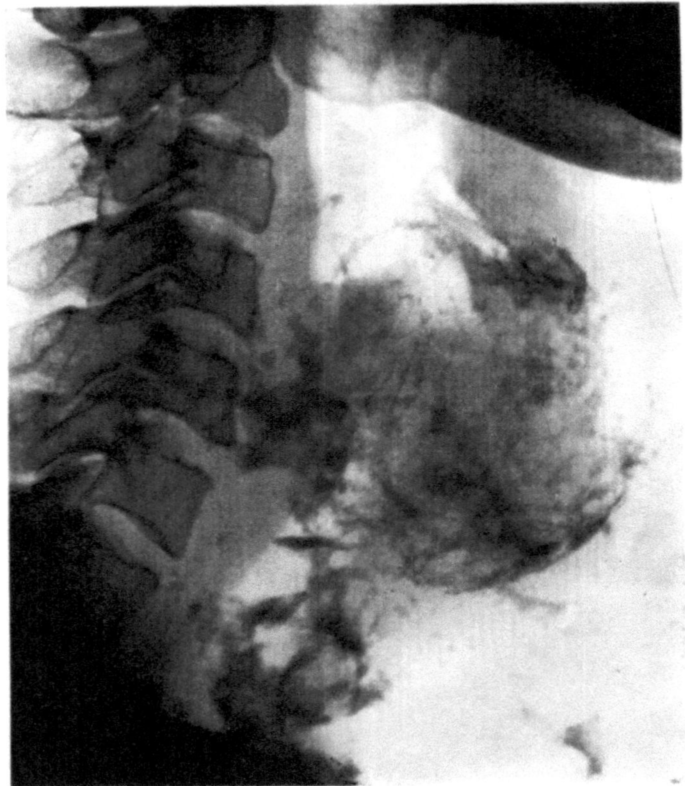

Fig. 155 Lateral view of the neck.

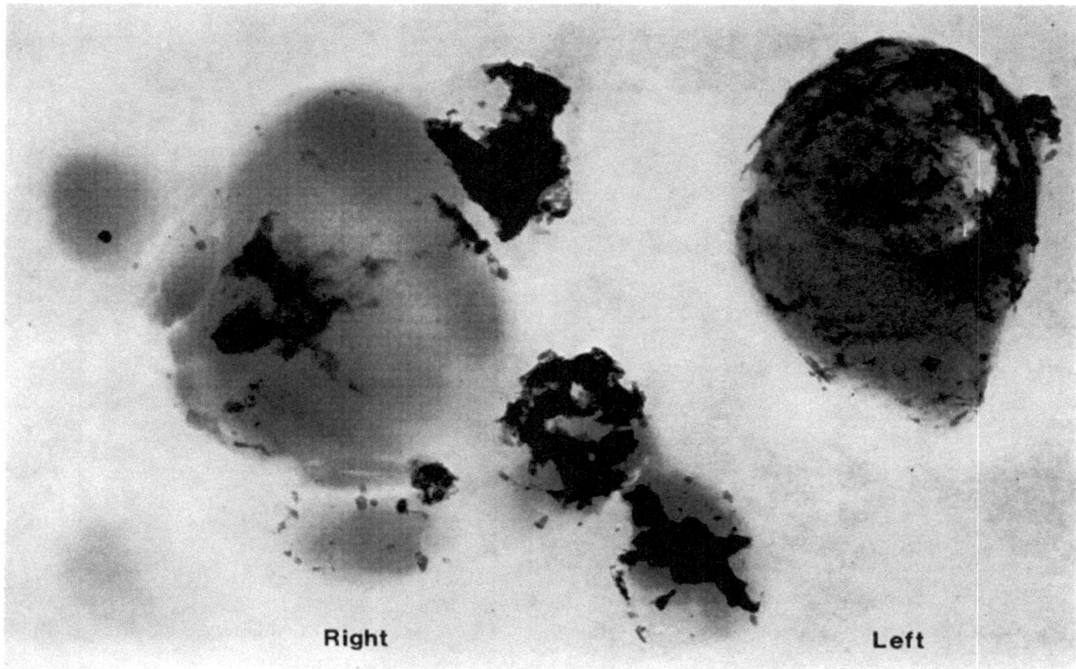

Fig. 156   Roentgenogram of the resected specimen.

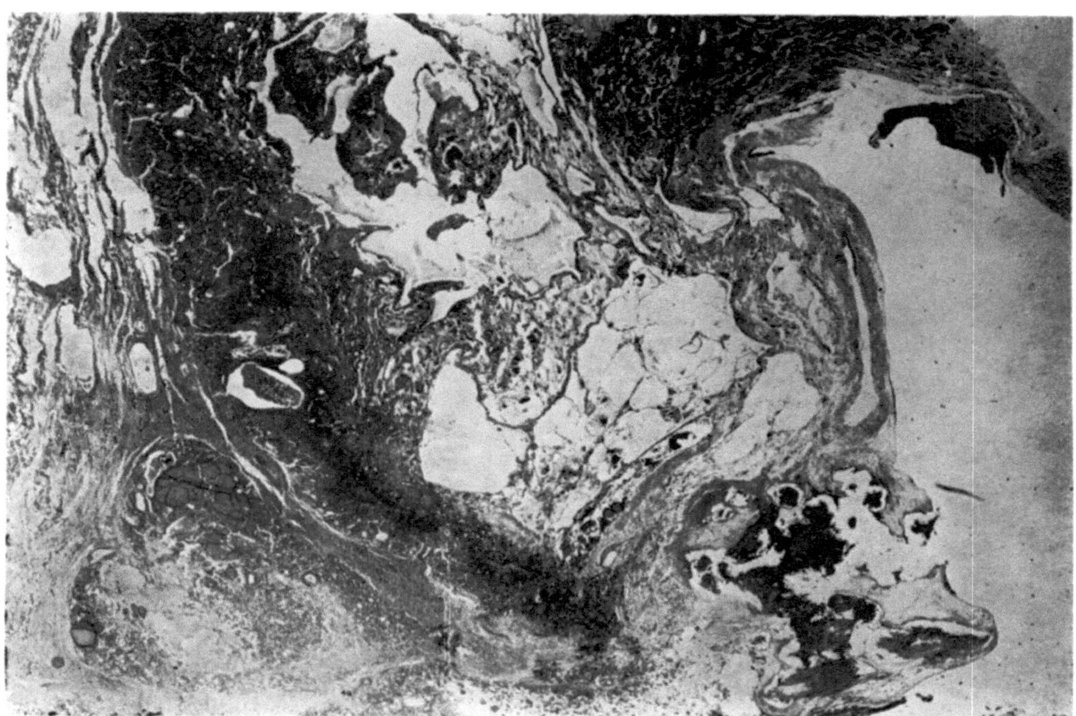

Fig. 157   Microscopic appearance, showing adenomatous growths.   Massive fibrosis occurred irregularly in the nodules, and the central portions of most of the nodules had undergone cystic degeneration.   (H & E, $\times$ 7)

REFERENCES

AKISADA, M. and FUJIMOTO, Y.: Soft tissue-spot-tangenital roentgenography in diagnosis of thyroid carcinoma—a method for detecting psammoma bodies. Nippon Acta Radiol., **31,** 1071, 1972.

AKISADA, M., WATANABE, H. and IKUSE, J.: Mammography (Part III). The fundamental studies and the significance of the microcalcifications of the breast carcinoma. Nippon Acta Radiol., **25,** 399, 1966. (in Japanese)

BATSAKIS, J. G., NISHIYAMA, R. H. and RICH, C. R.: Microlithiasis (calcospherites) and carcinoma of thyroid gland. Arch. Path., **69,** 493, 1960.

BOBBIO, A., BEZZI, E., ZANELLA, E. and ROSSI, L.: Angiographic aspects of disease of the thyroid. An evaluation of subclavian retrograde arteriographic procedures as a means of clinical study. J. Internat. Coll. Surgeons, **32,** 79, 1959.

CRILE, G., Jr. and FISHER, E. R.: Simultaneous occurence of thyroiditis and papillary carcinoma. Report of two cases. Cancer, **6,** 57, 1953.

DJINDJIAN, R. and DORLAND, P.: Arteriographie du corps thyroïde. J. radiol. électrol. méd. nucléaire, **44,** 605, 1963.

EGAN, R. L.: Mammography, p. 64, p. 75, Charles C Thomas Publisher, Springfield, Illinois, 1964.

ENDO, T., WATANABE, I., UMEZU, M., SHASHOKU, K., MATSUURA, K. and ISHII, S.: Arteriography of the thyroid galnd, with special refernce to the diagnosis of thyroid cancer. J. Japan. Surg. Soc., **69,** 1342, 1968. (in Japanese)

ERAZO, S. T. and WAHNER, H. W.: Roentgenographic diagnosis of thyroid cancer in the presence of endemic goiter. Amer. J. Roentgenol., Rad. Therapy & Nuclear Med., **96,** 596, 1966.

FOURNIER, A. M. and JOUVE-FOURNIER, P.: Considérations sur les calcifications thyroïdiennes. J. radiol. électrol. méd. nucléaire, **43,** 502, 1962.

FUJIMOTO, Y. and AKISADA, M.: Roentgenographic-histologic patterns of calcification in thyroid nodules. Endocrinol. Japan., **17,** 263, 1970.

FUJIMOTO, Y., OKA, A., OMOTO, R. and HIROSE, M.: Ultrasound scanning of the thyroid gland as as a new diagnostic approach. Ultrasonics, **5,** 177, 1967.

GASQUET, C. GÉRALD-MARCHANT, R., MARKOVITS, P. et TUBIANA, M.: Intérêt respectif du radio-diagnostic et la gammagraphie pour le diagnostic des cancers thyroïdiens. Bulletin du Cancer, **50,** 347, 1963.

GÉRALD-MARCHANT, R., PICARD, J. D., BABINET, J. et GASQUET, C.: Les calcifications thyroïdilennes, valeur diagnostique. Presse méd., 70, 1849, 1962.

GERSHON-COHEN, J. and HERMEL, M. B.: Advances in mammographic technique. Amer. J. Roentgenol., Rad. Therapy & Nuclear Med., **108,** 424, 1970.

GROS, C. H.: Méthodologie. J. radiol. électrol. méd. nucléaire, **48,** 638. 1967.

HIGUCHI, K., HORIE, H., NODA, T., FURUIZUMI, K., ASANAGI, S., ARAI, Y., HANADA, Y., AOKI, R. and HOSHI, S.: Diagnosis and therapy of thyroid cancer. Iryo, **23,** 10, 1969. (in Japanese)

HISADA, T., HIGUCHI, K. and YAMAGUCHI, T.: Clinico-pathological studies on the thyroid nodules. Folia Endocrinol. Japon., **38,** 261, 1962. (in Japanese)

HOLTZ, S. and POWERS, W. E.: Calcification in papillary carcinoma of thyroid. Amer. J. Roentgenol., Rad. Therapy & Nuclear Med., **80,** 997, 1958.

HOSHI, S., HIGUCHI, K. and HORIE, H.: Histopathological studies on the calcifications in the thyroid nodules. Iryo, **21,** 26, 1967 (in Japanese)

ITO, K., HIGASHI, Y., NISHIKAWA, Y., SEKIYA, M., KOMORI, A., MATSUDAIRA, H. and OYAMADA, H.: Differentiation between benign and malignant thyroid nodules based on roentgenographic patterns of calcification. Rinsho Hoshasen (Clin. Radiol.), **10,** 118, 1965. (in Japanese)

Ito, K., Nishikawa, Y., Harada, T., Suzuki, T. and Higashi, Y.: Roentgenologic examination of thyroid tumors. Clin. Endocrinol., **17**, 711, 1969. (in Japanese)

Klinck, G. H., Jr.: Papillary tumors of thyroid gland. New York J. Med., **49**, 302, 1949.

Klinck, G. H., Jr. and Winship, T.: Psammoma bodies and thyroid cancer. Cancer, **12**, 656, 1959.

Margolin, F. R. and Steinbach, H. L.: Soft tissue roentgenography of thyroid nodules. Amer. J. Roentgenol., Rad. Therapy & Nuclear Med., **102**, 844, 1968.

Margolin, F. R., Winfield, J. and Steinbach, H. L.: Patterns of thyroid calcification: Roentgenologic-histologic study of excised specimens. Invest. Radiol., **2**, 208, 1967.

Maruchi, N., Furihata, R. and Makiuchi, M.: Population surveys on the prevalence of thyroid cancer in a non-endemic region, Nagano, Japan. Internat. J. Cancer, **7**, 575, 1971.

Matoba, N. and Kikuchi, T.: Thyroidolymphography. A new technic for visualization of the thyroid and cervical lymph nodes. Radiology, **92**, 339, 1969.

Mittermaier, R.: Otorhinolaryngologic Radiology. A Radiologic Atlas of Ear, Nose and Throat Diseases, p. 196, Georg Thieme, Stuttgart, 1970. (English edition)

Onishi, S.: Calcification and bony metaplasia of the thyroid. Geka (Surgery), **28**, 876, 1966. (in Japanese)

Payr, E. and Matina, A.: Über wahre laterale Nebenkröpfe; Pathologisch-anatomische und klinische Beiträge. Deutsche Ztschr. Chir., **85**, 535, 1906.

Ritvo, M.: Chest X-ray Diagnosis, p. 412. Lea & Febiger, Philadelphia, 1951.

Scheier, M.: Über die Ossification des Kehlkopfs. Arch. mikr. Anat., **95**, 220, 1901.

Schein, C., Lentino, W. and Jacobson, H. G.: Relation of thyroid enlargement to tracheal configulation. Anatomico-roentgenologic correlation. New Eng. J. Med., **255**, 1072, 1956.

Segal, R. L., Zuckerman, H. and Friedman, E. W.: Soft tissue roentgenography: Its use in diagnosis of thyroid carcinoma. J.A.M.A., **173**, 1890, 1960.

Stanton, L. and Lightfoot, D. A.: Obtaining proper contrast in mammography. Radiology, **87**, 111, 1966.

Takahashi, M., Ishibashi, T. and Kawanami, H.: Angiographic diagnosis of benign and malignant tumors of the thyroid. Radiology, **92**, 520, 1969.

Thijs, L. G.: Diagnostic ultrasound in clinical thyroid investigation. J. Clin. Endocrinol., **32**, 709, 1971.

Underwood, C. R., Ackerman, L. U. and Eckert, C.: Papillary carcinoma of thyroid; Evaluation of surgical therapy. Surgery, **43**, 610, 1958.

Watanabe, T., Makiuchi, M., Sato, T. and Furihata, R.: Roentgenologic studies on the thyroid nodules: I. Patterns of calcification. Folia Endocrinol. Japon., **45**, 1471, 1970. (in Japanese)

INDEX

Page numbers in bold face indicate main discussions of the topics

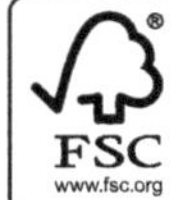